Geriatric Medicine

Geriatric Medicine

300 Specialty Certificate Exam Questions

By

Dr Shibley Rahman

Special advisor, NHS Practitioner Health,
Riverside Medical Centre, St George Wharf,
Wandsworth Road, London
Honorary research fellow, UCL Institute
of Cardiovascular Science, London

Dr Henry J. Woodford

Consultant Geriatrician, Northumbria Healthcare,
North Tyneside General Hospital

Forewords by
Professor Adam Gordon
and Professor Michael Vassallo

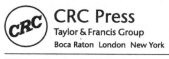

CRC Press

Taylor & Francis Group
Boca Raton London New York

CRC Press is an imprint of the
Taylor & Francis Group, an **informa** business

First edition published 2022
by CRC Press
6000 Broken Sound Parkway NW, Suite 300, Boca Raton, FL 33487–2742

and by CRC Press
2 Park Square, Milton Park, Abingdon, Oxon, OX14 4RN

© 2022 Taylor & Francis Group, LLC

CRC Press is an imprint of Taylor & Francis Group, LLC

ISBN: 978-0-367-56402-5 (hbk)
ISBN: 978-0-367-56400-1 (pbk)
ISBN: 978-1-003-09755-6 (ebk)

Typeset in Times
by Apex CoVantage, LLC

Contents

Foreword by Professor Adam Gordon

Effective care for older people lies at the heart of modern healthcare delivery. Rapid population ageing around the globe has seen a shift in the age distribution of patients that present to healthcare practitioners. Most acute hospital takes, or clinic lists, regardless of specialty, are increasingly filled by older people with multiple complex long-term conditions and/or frailty and/or disability and/or cognitive impairment.

This has challenged the traditional medical diagnostic paradigm. The process of establishing differential diagnoses, ruling things in or out through tests, and initiating curative treatments doesn't hold true in the face of multiple long-term conditions that interact in a multifactorial way to present as atypical geriatric syndromes. The evidence-based approach here is comprehensive geriatric assessment—a multi-domain, multi-professional, assessment-driven approach to build person-centred problem lists that drive case management.

Comprehensive geriatric assessment has a compelling evidence base. Randomised controlled trials that compare it with traditional models of care show that patients managed in this way have better functional and cognitive outcomes and lower mortality. But delivering, and leading, comprehensive geriatric assessment requires broad competencies, ranging from subspecialty expertise in common presentations in older people to an understanding of rehabilitation, palliative care, mental health, and how multidisciplinary teams can interact under each of these headings to deliver evidence-based gold-standard care.

The growing specialty of geriatric medicine has such competencies at its core. Substantial work has been undertaken over the last decade to establish expert consensus around core competencies in geriatric medicine and to lay them out in ways that they can be easily taught and learned. In the UK, where geriatric medicine is well established and is, in fact, the largest of the physicianly specialties, assessments have been added to higher specialty training to ensure that those who are eligible to become geriatricians have demonstrated these competencies. The Specialty Certificate Examination (SCE) tests the knowledge components of these competencies.

Building an SCE is, in fact, a long, highly structured and quality-controlled process. It starts with the higher specialty training curriculum, developed through expert consensus and honed over years of drafting and redrafting. Questions are written by specialists in the field against the learning outcomes included in the curriculum and then undergo multiple iterations and stages of quality control to ensure that they are unambiguous and correct. Finally, they are integrated into an exam in a way that covers a sufficient breadth of the curriculum.

Producing a textbook to emulate the SCE is no small feat. With this volume, Drs Rahman and Woodford have done a superb job. They have mirrored the processes of blueprinting, drafting and quality control that take place in the exam preparation processes for SCE under the stewardship of the Royal Colleges. It is also impressive that they have taken time to outline these processes, so that candidates can understand both how questions are derived and the rigour that goes into preparing the assessment process.

The authors emulate the 'single best answer' of the SCE examination. This is peculiarly well suited to geriatric medicine. The point of a single best answer question is to test not just knowledge but also judgement. It is usually the case that more than one answer is partially correct. This, as a practising geriatrician, is the decisional challenge that I face on a daily basis. Multiple diagnoses, multiple investigations and multiple management plans, and combinations upon combinations of these, represent a panoply of possibilities for the attending physician. This format is good not just because it emulates what is used in the exam. It is good because it hones exactly the sort of decisional competencies required to be a good geriatrician.

Within the topics listed are some things that are difficult to test, including questions around rehabilitation and transfers of care. The challenge here is usually to recognise what is required of doctors, and how their contributions interdigitate with the multiple other professionals required to deliver care for older people. The authors have captured this well. Rehabilitation does not start and end with the input of the geriatrician—but a geriatrician's input can be valuable, particularly if informed by the types of expertise that the questions here will help hone.

The questions here will be, of course, an invaluable resource to future geriatricians preparing for the SCE. They will be useful for geriatricians from outside the UK who want to hone and benchmark their knowledge against the curricular outcomes included in one of the very few

higher specialty progress examinations for geriatricians internationally. There's also useful learning here for other hospital specialists, for general practitioners, for nurses and for allied health professionals who want to build their knowledge around care of older people. There will never be enough geriatricians—other healthcare professionals will find their jobs much easier, and more rewarding, if they bank the knowledge included in these pages.

It's important to realise that the SCE covers only the knowledge-based components of progress assessment in higher specialty training. Geriatric medicine is, though, a very hands-on specialty. Our British trainees demonstrate the prerequisite skills and attitudes through a series of workplace-based assessments. Most geriatricians choose their specialty because they enjoy the intellectual challenge of managing complexity and uncertainty, but it is in our interactions with our patients that geriatric medicine comes to life. Drs Rahman and Woodford are commended for breathing life and verisimilitude into the clinical scenarios in this book. If you're a geriatrician and, having worked through these problems, you feel the urge to get back on the wards, then you've chosen the correct specialty. If you're not a geriatrician, and you feel the same urge, then you've become part of the revolution that promises to deliver the care that patients attending healthcare services actually need. Welcome. *Vive la révolution!*

Adam Gordon
Professor of Care of Older People,
University of Nottingham
President-Elect, British Geriatrics
Society
January 2021

Foreword by Michael Vassallo

The specialty certificate exam (SCE) in geriatric medicine has been developed as an assessment of knowledge and is an important high-stakes landmark in the training of specialist trainees in geriatric medicine in the United Kingdom. It is an essential requirement for the completion of training and without it, trainees cannot gain entry into the specialist register held by the General Medical Council (GMC). Passing the exam demonstrates that the candidate has the knowledge required to be able to work as a consultant in the United Kingdom. Since opening up the exam to candidates outside of training programmes, interest has also grown amongst non-trainees nationally and internationally. I was chair of the exam board for seven years and secretary for three years before that, working with my predecessor Oliver Corrado, who led in setting it up and to whom I pay tribute. I can confirm that the need to prepare for the exam cannot be understated. Prospective candidates must study and prepare for it, as the knowledge acquired from day-to-day routine work is unlikely to be enough to successfully pass the exam without additional reading. For this reason there is an ongoing need for educational material to support preparation by prospective candidates. Such material needs to be current and reflective of the rapidly changing evidence-based practice in geriatric medicine that has characterised the last decade. In my opinion the book *Geriatric Medicine: 300 Specialty Certificate Exam Questions* written by Dr Shibley Rahman and Dr Henry J. Woodford is a very useful and timely addition to the educational material available to prepare for the exam.

It is an extremely well-written comprehensive text that covers all aspects of the preparation required from prospective candidates. It is not just a collection of questions but offers many useful tips about the preparation required. In their preface the authors clearly and logically explain the rationale behind setting up the exam. They direct candidates to additional useful reading material when preparing for the exam as well as include a number of very useful links to key official documents such as the blueprint and curriculum. They explain how the exam is developed and standard set, giving insight into the complex process of making the paper. Importantly they provide various very helpful tips about examination technique. This I feel is a crucial and sometimes missed aspect of the preparation. As previous chair of the exam board, it used to distress me considerably hearing about trainees being turned away from the exam centre because they arrived ten minutes late or because they did not have the correct identification to allow entry. It is such a shame that all that preparation and expense involved is lost for such trivial reasons, not to mention the impact on career progression. I would therefore like to emphasise the points made by the authors to very carefully read the instructions sent before the exam and make sure you arrive early. Consider staying overnight if you have to travel far. It is a very long day—you must conserve your mental energy for when you need it to deliver. On such an important day one must not leave any stone unturned, always bearing in mind Murphy's law, 'if it can go wrong it will'.

True to the format of the exam, the authors write 300 best of five questions in a collection of chapters based on blueprint headings. The blueprint is an important document as it determines the format of the paper and the number of questions for each section the candidate can expect. In these various chapters the authors proportionately follow the contents of the blueprint. This supports the candidate in using time judiciously to avoid spending a disproportionate amount of reading on an area of the curriculum where the number of questions is going to be limited. Time management is an important aspect of the preparation of this exam. In the various chapters, the authors present clear learning objectives followed by a series of best of five questions, which is the format used in the exam itself. In such questions the candidate is likely to find a number of plausible answers, and the aim is to find the best single answer. This is not easy and often requires decisions based on experience. The scenarios presented in the questions are very well chosen to reflect real-time geriatric medicine, and this is a credit to the authors' experience. Several questions require a situational judgement to be made. This reproduces that everyday feeling of needing to think on your feet when it comes to providing solutions to the complex presentations one sees in clinical practice. They cover all the topics tested in the exam, including acute and chronic internal medicine, dementia and delirium, continence, falls, comprehensive geriatric assessment, stroke, nutrition, old age psychiatry, and other specialty topics such as surgical liaison and orthogeriatrics. Each chapter is concluded with answers that explain the rationale behind the correct answer with appropriate readings that inform this. Readings include textbooks, peer-reviewed high-impact journals and the latest guidelines. This shows the meticulous approach taken by the authors in writing the text. The candidates preparing for the exam can be assured of the quality of the answers given.

Finally, although this text has been written for doctors in training programmes preparing for the SCE, it is also a valuable aid for those sitting other exams on a similar format such as the Diploma in Geriatric Medicine. However, the book is fundamentally about geriatric medicine and about real scenarios from day-to-day clinical work. It is therefore also valuable to established geriatricians as well as other members of the multidisciplinary team who want to keep themselves up to date.

The style of the text is easy to read, and the scenarios raised in the questions will resonate with all interested adult learners working in elderly medicine. This is a book that I thoroughly recommend. It has a good mix of easy and difficult questions pitched at the level one would expect at the SCE. I really enjoyed reading it and I felt I learnt a lot, and it is excellent preparation for the SCE and other written exams in geriatric medicine.

Prof Michael Vassallo
MD FRCP (Lond) FRCP (Edin), DGM, PhD, MPhil, FAcadMEd
Consultant Physician
Director of Medical Education
Visiting Professor Bournemouth University
Vice President for Education and Training British Geriatrics Society
February 2021

Acknowledgments

The authors should like to offer genuine and sincere thanks to Prof Adam Gordon, President-Elect of the British Geriatrics Society, for the Foreword to this book, and to Dr Clifford Lisk for offering constructive criticism on these questions and answers, as an experienced consultant geriatrician and medical educator. Finally, both the authors would like to acknowledge the significant contribution made by Prof Michael Vassallo to education and training of the workforce in geriatric medicine and to the initial development of the SCE exam.

About the Authors

Dr Shibley Rahman was born in Glasgow and trained in medicine at Cambridge University, where he also completed his PhD in the neurocognition of frontotemporal dementia. He also trained in international law and business management from London to postgraduate level. He is currently employed as special advisor in disability at the NHS Practitioner Health. He has research interests in dementia, delirium and frailty, and is a member of the special interest groups of the European Geriatric Medical Society in dementia and delirium. Other publications include *Living Well with Dementia*, which won BMJ best of the book award in 2015. Outside of formal work, he is a family carer and interested in cooking. He posts occasionally on Twitter (@ dr_shibley).

Dr Henry J. Woodford was born in York but completed his training in medicine at King's College London. He is currently employed as a consultant geriatrician at Northumbria Healthcare in the northeast of England. He has a particular interest in medicines optimisation for older people and is chair of the relevant British Geriatrics Society special interest group. Other publications include the textbook *Essential Geriatrics*. Outside of work, he tries to keep fit through circuit training, running and indoor bouldering. He posts occasionally on Twitter, including the cartoon strip 'the Wholly Frail' (@woodford_henry).

Introduction

This book is intended to be a positive learning experience in itself.

The aim of our text is to have a closer look at the full range of the topics in the Specialty Certificate Examination (SCE) for geriatric medicine and to offer a selection of 300 questions to reflect the knowledge, giving coverage to reflect the 'blueprint', and the current geriatric training curriculum from Joint Royal Colleges of Physicians Training Board (JRCPTB).

Most UK trainees pass the exam. Trainees have a vast amount of experience from their 'routine' clinical work.

About the SCE and Postgraduate Medical Exams

It is worth us first demystifying some elements of this assessment.

Learning depends on many interrelated factors, including those related to the student, the educator, the curriculum and the environment within which learning takes place. There is now a drive away from curricula that dissuade students from simple 'rote learning' and a drive towards curricula that encourage deep processing.

The curriculum is a statement of the intended aims and objectives, content, experiences, outcomes and processes of a programme, and the assessment is a systematic procedure for measuring a trainee's progress or level of achievement against defined criteria.

There are currently no entry requirements for the SCE in geriatric medicine, although candidates in UK training posts should have taken the SCE by the end of training year ST5, towards Certificate of Completion of Training (CCT) and Annual Review of Competency Progression (ARCP). It is not intended to act as a barrier to your career progression.

You should be approaching this test in a calm and strategic manner.

There are no 'trick questions'. There are no intentional 'red herrings'. The examiners on behalf of the College are not trying to trick you. This means that, if a question looks easy, it is an easy question. Take the questions at face value. If it looks easy, it probably is.

The SCE is a summative assessment of scientific and clinical knowledge, as well as problem-solving ability. It is a national-level assessment run by the RCP, equivalent to subspecialty exams from North America, and is likewise important for public confidence. It is supposed to confer the status of a 'certified specialist' in terms of theory and works in conjunction with work-based assessments. It is therefore a quality assurance too. It covers all areas of knowledge that you should have acquired during your specialty training. It gives the public confidence that consultants have the right level of knowledge.

Curricula for the medical specialties are available from the JRCPTB website (www.jrcptb.org.uk). Preparation for the SCE requires a wide breadth of knowledge around the curriculum and should involve the reading of up-to-date textbooks, journals and guidelines. National Institute for Health and Care Excellence (NICE) guidance is useful; not necessarily the full guidance, but the summary documents at least (e.g. hypertension, heart failure, continence, stroke, dementia, delirium). Whilst explanations in this book refer to guidance, you should always get hold of and consult the up-to-date version of the guidance, which might have changed subsequent to publication of this book. Get familiar with screening tools, such as in cognition, nutrition and osteoporosis. Experience of the MRCP(UK) examination provides an excellent background to the format of the examination, including geriatric questions in MRCP question banks. A way to approach your preparation does not include a detailed or an in-depth study of a large geriatrics textbook. Finally, there is huge value in knowledge and judgement arising from your vast clinical experience on the wards until and including this point in your training.

Candidates are advised to attempt the SCE for the first time towards the end of their specialist medical training, by which time they are likely to have acquired the breadth of experience necessary for familiarity with the clinical scenarios used in the questions. However, there are no restrictions on when you may make your first attempt, and it is no longer necessary for applicants for the SCE in any specialty to have passed the MRCP(UK) examination. Practicing as many exam questions as possible is an effective study strategy, and you can find example questions on the MRCP(UK) website. Effective exam technique is important.

The geriatric medicine SCE tests the 'knowledge' part of the geriatric medicine curriculum—but not the content of your everyday work. This is an important distinction to understand. You may instinctively answer the question based on your clinical experience, which may not lead you to the 'correct' answer. You therefore need to read the syllabus section of the curriculum, which can be found on the JRCPTB website. You also need to be conversant in the details of current

relevant guidelines. The exam will be faithful to reliable sources of medical guidance, such as NICE guidelines or the major societies. For example, by studying carefully, the JRCPTB curriculum is likely to enrich your enjoyment of your clinical practice and to motivate you to find out more about contemporary geriatrics from international societies such as the British Geriatrics Society (BGS). The BGS is very keen to offer an annual workshop to prepare trainees and other students for the SCE examination and has now done so for many years.

Postgraduate curricula and assessments are implemented so that doctors in training are able to demonstrate what is expected in good medical practice and to achieve the learning outcomes required by their curriculum. Postgraduate deaneries and medical schools make sure that medical education and training take place in an environment and culture that meets these standards, within their own organisation and through effective quality management of contracts, agreements and local quality control mechanisms. They work together to respond when patient safety and training concerns are associated. Overall, this provides a base of knowledge acceptable to the UK medical regulator, the General Medical Council (GMC).

'Promoting Excellence: Standards for Medical Education and Training' is, for example, a GMC document which sets out ten standards that the GMC expects organisations responsible for educating and training medical students and doctors in the UK to meet. The standards and requirements are organised around five themes. Some requirements—what an organisation must do to show the GMC they are meeting the standards—may apply to a specific stage of education and training.

The Federation of Royal Colleges of Physicians of the United Kingdom is a collection of three professional bodies (Royal College of Physicians of Edinburgh, Royal College of Physicians and Surgeons of Glasgow and Royal College of Physicians London) which aims to improve the quality of patient care by continually raising medical standards. Launched in 2008, SCEs from the Federation of Royal Colleges of Physicians of the United Kingdom were proposed to articulate the 'gold standard' postgraduate qualification for physicians looking to progress in their specialty. They provide the opportunity to measure a level of knowledge against an 'internationally recognised yardstick', which represents the breadth and depth of knowledge required of a newly qualified specialist in your chosen discipline.

The SCEs are currently run in various different specialities and are designed to test specialist knowledge as trainees reach the end of their training programme. The SCEs assess knowledge and understanding of the clinical sciences relevant to specialist medical practice and of common or important disorders to a level appropriate for a newly appointed consultant. They also provide a professional standard against which physicians working outside the UK can measure their level of attainment.

It is envisaged that international doctors will sit this exam either after having obtained MRCP(UK) or as they near the end of their training. The problem with setting the examination is that jurisdiction-specific knowledge, such as law relating to older patients or welfare benefits, poses assessment difficulties.

Blueprint, Curriculum and 'Standard Setting'

Exam 'blueprinting' is a method which achieves valid assessment of students by defining exactly what is intended to be measured in which learning domain and defines what level of competence is required.

The exam reflects that the field is geriatric medicine, not simply general internal medicine in older people.

No standard-setting method can yield an 'optimal' cut-score value as this is determined by the experts' internal construction of what constitutes competence. The primary use of any test score in a criterion-referenced setting is to determine whether a candidate has mastered a set of competencies presumed to underlie performance on the examination. Specialists may therefore advise on what borderline candidates would be expected to answer correctly at a minimum. The Angoff standard-setting approach is one of the most widely used in medicine. Certain questions are going to be tougher, with a varying percentage of candidates getting them right. The pass mark remains roughly consistent every year, and the performance of questions is statistically reviewed every year to ensure standards are consistent. Standard setting for the MRCP(UK) examinations, in which the SCE might be considered a member of the family, has traditionally used a hybrid of the Angoff and Hofstede methods. The pass mark is specific to a diet of the examination, depending on the actual questions in the examination. There is no 'arbitrary' pass mark.

In its purest form, the Angoff method is a judgemental approach in which a group of expert judges makes estimates about how borderline candidates would perform on items in the examination, that is, the proportion of borderline examinees who will answer an item correctly. Another method is the 'classical Hofstede method' where judges decide on the minimum and maximum failure rate and acceptable pass mark. But recent research has found that an effective method of standard setting is 'statistical equating' using item response theory (McManus et al., 2014).

None of the contributors to this book have ever been members of the Standard Setting or Question Writing Group for the SCE proper. Members of the Standard Setting Group advise on the pass mark to be applied to the examination paper. Members of this group are responsible for evaluating the level of difficulty of each question in an examination paper in order to set a pass mark; ensuring that the quality of individual questions is high and that the examination questions are of an appropriate standard; and keeping abreast of developments in the world of medical education and medical practice, ensuring that the examination papers are relevant to the curriculum. It is important that actual participants in the SCE setting process have considerable knowledge of the examination, have experience of standard setting and question writing in an academic environment and understand the statistical methods and principles used commonly in standard setting and interpretation of analyses performed on individual items.

Current links to key official documents:

Blueprint—

www.mrcpuk.org/sites/default/files/
documents/sce-geriatric-medicine-
blueprint_01.pdf

Curriculum—

www.jrcptb.org.uk/sites/default/files/
2010%20Geriatric%20Medicine%
20Curriculum%20%28AMEND
MENTS%202016%29.pdf

There is scope for interpretation of these documents taken together. To enable an adequate coverage of pervasive themes such as medicines optimisation, frailty and movement disorders, for example, which are important in geriatric training and for success as a geriatric medicine specialist, there needs to be coverage of

these topics in the exam in suitable sections of the blueprint.

There is an exam blueprint that describes how many questions from each subject area will be included in the exam. This ensures that the entire curriculum is sampled. It is anticipated that this blueprint will be updated regularly to reflect the changing demands and needs of the higher specialist curriculum. The exam currently consists of two papers, each consisting of 100 'single best answer' (SBA) type (also known as 'best of five' type) questions. These may be on any subject contained within the geriatric medicine curriculum. There is some repetition of topics across the subsections of the curriculum. Subjects such as delirium, frailty, medicines optimisation, movement disorders, palliative care, age-related physiological changes and rehabilitation can appear in multiple areas. We have had to make what we feel are reasonable decisions to divide the knowledge to be assessed into the appropriate SCE sections and with the right number of questions overall.

The candidate is expected to display a level of knowledge equivalent to a consultant practising in geriatric medicine. This includes knowledge of basic science and gerontology, clinical scenarios and relevant guidelines and scoring systems. The overall number of questions on basic science and gerontology is quite small, so it is not worth worrying about them overly. The most clinically applicable SBA questions present a scenario, with relevant and plausible options (at least to the mind of a borderline candidate); the 'best' answer might be judged as 80% correct and the distractors perhaps 20%–30% correct. While students in clinical practice obviously do not have the prompt of possible options, SBAs do encourage students to work with conditional probabilities that compare to real clinical practice (Walsh et al., 2017).

Questions avoided in the question bank as far as possible are those which refer to highly specific numerical answers, but, where they exist, concern information which really ought to be known by the majority of higher specialist trainees.

The Format

Like most multiple choice test problems, once you know the content, the real issue is the test format itself. Multiple choice questions are a different way of looking at the material compared to how you learned it, and that's tricky for some people. You need to do as many sample multiple choice tests and questions as possible in the time leading up to the SCE.

The SCE is a computer-based, multiple choice test divided into two papers. Candidates are allowed three hours to answer each paper, which comprises 100 items. This means there are 108 seconds to answer each question roughly, except some questions are very short and take far fewer seconds. Each question presents a clinical scenario, with the results of some investigations and perhaps an image or scan, and tests your medical knowledge and your competency in diagnosis, investigation, management and prognosis. The College will be very grateful for your feedback.

SBA (or 'best of five') questions are widely used in undergraduate and postgraduate medical examinations. The typical format is a question stem describing a clinical vignette, followed by a lead-in question about the described scenario such as the likely diagnosis or the next step in the management plan. The candidate is presented with a list of possible responses and asked to choose the single best answer (Sam et al., 2016). All the options are plausible. One of the options is much more plausible and accurate than the others are. Some of the options are false altogether.

The questions which have been written and which are in the question bank have been set by well-rounded active clinical geriatricians with great care and argued over before being accepted on the bank. All questions which are banked have a consensus agreement about the answer.

The format of the SCE is based on the MRCP(UK) model and features:

- Two three-hour papers of 100 questions each.
- One annual diet per specialty.
- Electronic test taken on a computer at an official testing centre.

The test is taken at an independently operated assessment centre. These centres run in most countries.

Standards

The Federation of the Royal Colleges of Physicians set out the standards which apply to assessment of their training curricula, including the MRCP(UK) and SCE. It is worth noting that representatives of the BGS have a 'say' in the updating of the JRCPTB curriculum in geriatric medicine.

They are summarised as follows.

Examination Technique

The examination takes place in professional test centres, at the time of publication by PearsonVue. Some centres do not have parking facilities or places to buy lunch, so research your centre in advance.

Arrive in good time before the exam starts, and make sure you plan how to get to the test centre. Make sure you bring the correct official identification

TABLE 0.1

Based on Information Provided by the RCP London, the 'Standards' of the SCE Assessment.*

Standard number	Standard description	Application to SCE
2	The overall purpose of the assessment system must be documented and in the public domain.	The functions of each and all components of the SCE examination available to trainees, educators, employers, professional bodies, including the regulatory bodies, and the public.
3	The curriculum must set out the general, professional and specialty-specific content.	The relevant curriculum is the specialty curriculum in geriatric medicine.
4	Assessments must systematically sample the entire content and be appropriate to the stage of training, with reading to the common and important clinical problems that the trainee will encounter in the workplace.	Questions in the SCE sample the content of the relevant specialty curriculum.
5	Indication should be given of how curriculum implementation will be managed and assured locally and within approved programmes.	The JRCPTB is responsible for producing the UK medical specialty curricula. The RCP takes quality improvement very seriously.
8	The choice of assessment method(s) should be appropriate to the content and purpose of that element of the curriculum.	To test knowledge and application of knowledge in written examination 'best of five' multiple choice questions are used.
10	Assessors/examiners will be recruited against criteria for performing the tasks they undertake.	Guidance, induction and training are provided to new examiners specific to their rôle.
11	Assessments must provide relevant feedback to the trainees.	The RCP provides feedback to candidates following all of our examinations.
12	The methods used to set standards for classification of trainees' performance/ competence must be transparent and in the public domain.	Recognised methods to set the standards of the examination. As a result of the standard setting process, the pass mark and pass rate may vary at each SCE.
13	Documentation will record the results and consequences of assessments and the trainee's progress through the assessment system.	The results letters and certificates issued are standardised, and information on UK trainee examination performance is shared with the JRCPTB.
14	Plans for curriculum review, including curriculum evaluation and monitoring, must be set out.	The JRCPTB is responsible for ensuring that the UK medical specialty curricula remain up to date. The curriculum aims to respond quickly to new clinical and service developments. Trainees, patients and laypersons are involved in curricula review.
15	Resources and infrastructure will be available to support trainee learning and assessment.	The JRCPTB is responsible for producing the curricula, and each curriculum defines the process of training and the competencies required as well as how the curriculum was developed.
16	There will be lay and patient input in the development and implementation of assessments.	There is lay representation on the SCE Steering Group.

* Standards. www.mrcpuk.org/about-mrcpuk/academic-standards/standard-setting

documents to the exam, as this will be checked very carefully. You will need to prove that you have registered for the exam—check with current regulations. This is very important, as without the correct confirmatory documentation, it is not possible to sit the exam.

Other tests may be taking place simultaneously in the 'test room'—do not be put off by people leaving at a different time to you. The test centres provide water and secure lockers for the storage of candidates' belongings

You can't take *anything* into the assessment, but lockers are provided to keep your belongings safe.

There are specific rules about your attendance in the examination cubicle itself.

It's important to think about how you're going to answer the questions; here are some tips.

TABLE 0.2

Tips for Taking the SCE Assessment.

- After reading a question, try to summarise as precisely as possible, 'What is this question about ' and which part of the blueprint might it correspond to?'
- Try to answer the question *without* looking at the answer options.
- Then look at the answer options: you can usually narrow the correct answer down to two options.
- To decide which of the remaining options it could be, read the lead-in again carefully. For example: 'What is the most appropriate immediate treatment?' or 'What is the best diagnostic test to perform?' or 'What is the most likely diagnosis?'
- Finally, do not spend ages stuck on any one question. The worst thing you can do is spend a long time on a few and rush through the rest.

TABLE 0.3

Information Based on Current 'Blueprint'.*

Topic	Blueprint	This book
Acute illness (Diagnosis and Management)	29	44
Basic science and gerontology	6	9
Chronic disease and disability (Diagnosis and Management)	33	49
Cognitive impairment (Delirium and Dementia)	20	30
Continence	10	15
Falls and poor mobility	16	24
Geriatric assessment	8	12
Surgical liaison	3	5
Intermediate care and long-term care	9	13
Nutrition	4	6
Rehabilitation and transfers of care	14	21
Subspecialty topics: Palliative care	10	15
Subspecialty topics: Old age psychiatry	7	11
Subspecialty topics: Orthogeriatrics and osteoporosis	10	15
Subspecialty topics: Stroke care	15	22
Subspecialty topics: Tissue viability	6	9
Total	**200**	**300**

* Please check with original source, www.mrcpuk.org/sites/default/files/documents/sce-geriatric-medicine-blueprint_01.pdf.

SCE in Geriatric Medicine Blueprint

Candidates are tested on a wide range of common and important disorders as set out in the syllabus of the curriculum.

The composition of the paper is as follows (*correct at the time of publishing of this book, but please check with current specification*):

The questions in each category are distributed across both papers. Each chapter commences with the learning objectives and an extraction of key knowledge points from the JRCPTB curriculum in geriatric medicine.

Disclaimer: please do not rely on any part of this book as professional advice.

Best of luck.

Dr Shibley Rahman
London
Dr Henry J. Woodford
Northumberland
February 2021

READING

General

McManus IC, Chis L, Fox R, Waller D, Tang P. Implementing statistical equating for MRCP(UK) Parts 1 and 2. BMC Med Educ 2014; 14: 204.

Oxford Textbook of Medical Education. Ed. Kieran Walsh. Oxford: Oxford University Press, 2016.

Sam, AH, Hameed S, Harris J, et al. Validity of very short answer versus single best answer questions for undergraduate assessment. BMC Med Educ 2016; 16: 266.

Understanding medical education: Evidence, theory and practice (Third edition). Eds. Tim Swanwick, Kirsty Forrest, Bridget C. O'Brien. Oxford, UK: Wiley-Blackwell, 21 Dec, 2018.

Walsh JL, Harris BHL, Smith PE. Single best answer question-writing tips for clinicians. Postgrad Med J 2017; 93: 76–81.

RCP *Exams*

Specialty Certificate Examinations: Qualifications to broaden your horizons. www.mrcpuk.org/sites/default/files/documents/specialty-certificate-examinations-qualifications-to-broader-your-horizons.pdf.

Standards. www.mrcpuk.org/about-mrcpuk/academic-standards/standard-setting.

www.mrcpuk.org/mrcpuk-examinations/specialty-certificate-examinations/specialties/geriatric-medicine.

GMC

Promoting excellence: Standards for medical education and training. www.gmc-uk.org/education/standards-guidance-and-curricula/standards-and-outcomes/promoting-excellence.

Standards for curricula and assessment systems. www.gmc-uk.org/-/media/documents/Standards_for_curricula_and_assessment_systems_1114_superseded_0517.pdf_48904896.pdf.

1

Acute Illness (Diagnosis and Management)

LEARNING OBJECTIVE:

To be able to diagnose and manage acute illness and emergencies, including both medical and surgical conditions, in older patients across a variety of settings.

This might include emergency presentations across diverse conditions, including exacerbations of chronic diseases:

- Anaemia/haematology
- Cardiovascular medicine
- Dermatology
- Endocrine and metabolic medicine (including hypothermia and hyperthermia, neuroleptic malignant syndrome)
- Gastroenterology (including constipation, diarrhoea, faecal impaction)
- Infection and sepsis
- Musculoskeletal medicine (including physical deconditioning)
- Neurology
- Renal medicine (fluid/electrolyte imbalance)
- Respiratory medicine
- Sensory impairment

Other aspects might include:

- Drugs, including compliance, interactions and unwanted effects, in older people.

- Ethical and legal framework for making decisions on behalf of patients who lack mental capacity.
- Secondary complications of acute illness in older people and strategies to prevent them.
- Older people's physiological management.

Questions

Question 1

An 85-year-old man is admitted from his own home with pneumonia. He has a past history of cerebrovascular disease and vascular dementia. He has poor dental health, bi-basal chest crackles and an impaired swallow. It is suspected that he has developed pneumonia due to aspiration. Which of the following interventions has been shown to lower the risk of aspiration pneumonia in older people?

A. improved oral hygiene

B. percutaneous endoscopic gastrostomy tube feeding

C. physical exercise group activities

D. thickened fluids

E. using newer atypical antipsychotic drugs in preference to older typical ones

Question 2

You see a 92-year-old man acutely admitted to your ward with cellulitis of the left leg. As a coincidental discovery, he was found to have atrial fibrillation on his ECG. You are considering whether to offer him anticoagulation to reduce the risk of future embolic stroke but are cautious due to him having moderate to severe frailty. Which of the following is a component of the HAS-BLED score?

A. heart failure

B. high blood pressure

C. peptic ulcer disease

D. recent head injury

E. surgery within the last three months

Question 3

While on call you are phoned by a GP asking for help with the interpretation of a blood test result for a patient with suspected heart failure. Which of the following scenarios is more likely to result in an elevated serum N-terminal pro-B-type natriuretic peptide (NT-proBNP) concentration?

A. African or African-Caribbean family origin

B. age over 70 years

C. current ACE inhibitor use

D. current beta-blocker use

E. obesity

Question 4

A 73-year-old man has been admitted due to a fall on the background of a general decline in his physical and cognitive function over the last few weeks. His past history includes cerebrovascular disease, vascular dementia and depression. His usual medications are clopidogrel 75 mg od, atorvastatin 40 mg nocte, ramipril 5 mg od and solifenacin 5 mg od. While in hospital he was started on quetiapine for his agitation and mirtazapine for low mood. Over the last 24 hours he has been noted to be drowsier, and is not responding verbally at present. His temperature is 38.1°C, pulse 118 beats per minute and blood pressure 184/97 mmHg. Examination of his chest and abdomen are unremarkable. His pupils are 2 mm bilaterally and reactive to light, tone is increased in all of his limbs and reflexes appear normal. What is the most likely diagnosis?

A. anticholinergic toxicity

B. dementia with Lewy bodies

C. neuroleptic malignant syndrome

D. serotonin syndrome

E. urinary tract infection

Question 5

A 78-year-old woman has been admitted following a fall at home occurring while she was hurrying to get to the toilet during the night. She has a history of watery diarrhoea over the last four weeks, passing loose stools three to six times each day, including overnight. She has had several episodes of associated faecal incontinence. Three days prior to admission, she had a colonoscopy performed, which had not shown any macroscopic abnormalities (biopsy results awaited). Her GP had also sent a stool culture one week ago which had also not detected any abnormality. Blood tests show that she is mildly dehydrated but otherwise normal, including coeliac serology. Her past history includes ischaemic heart disease, hypertension and a cholecystectomy for gallstones. She takes aspirin 75 mg od, simvastatin 40 mg nocte and amlodipine 5 mg od. She normally lives alone and is independent in her personal care. Physical examination is unremarkable. Which investigation or action would be most appropriate to do next?

A. faecal calprotectin test

B. faecal elastase test

C. hydrogen breath test

D. ^{75}SeHCAT test

E. start oral budesonide

Question 6

A 71-year-old man presents with urinary incontinence and reduced mobility. Usually he is independently mobile and self-caring. He has a past history of type 2 diabetes and hypertension. He also has a many-year history of chronic back pain, which has been a little worse recently. A bladder scan shows >999 mL of urine within his bladder. His BMI is 35 kg/m^2 but he reports that he has lost some weight recently. On examination, his abdomen is soft and non-tender but there is fullness supra-pubically. His heart sounds are normal and his chest is clear. Sensation and power appear intact in his lower limbs, but his knee and ankle reflexes are diminished. Which investigation would you do next?

A. CT abdomen and pelvis

B. intravenous urogram

C. MRI spine

D. prostate specific antigen

E. urine culture

Question 7

A 77-year-old man has been admitted to hospital after having been found in a state of reduced responsiveness by his carer. Over the past week he had complained of a cough, and his oral intake had declined. He is found to be drowsy and looks clinically dehydrated. His past medical history includes type 2 diabetes that is controlled with a combination of metformin and twice daily insulin. There is no prior evidence of renal impairment. His observations show pulse 113 beats per minute, blood pressure 88/46 mmHg, respiratory rate 28 per minute, temperature 37.6°C and weight 79 kg.

TABLE 1.1

Investigations.

Serum sodium	159 mmol/L (137–144)
Serum potassium	5.2 mmol/L (3.5–4.9)
Random plasma glucose	41 mmol/L (4.0–7.8)
Serum urea	35.3 mmol/L (2.5–7.8)
Serum creatinine	216 μmol/L (64–104)
Serum osmolality	379 mOsm/L (285–295)
Chest X-ray	Right basal consolidation

He is commenced on intravenous antibiotics for pneumonia. In addition to this, which is the best initial treatment for this man?

A. 0.45% sodium chloride 1 L over one hour

B. 0.9% sodium chloride 1 L over one hour

C. 0.45% sodium chloride 1 L over one hour, plus insulin infusion at rate of four units per hour

D. 0.9% sodium chloride 1 L over one hour, plus insulin infusion at rate of four units per hour

E. 0.45% sodium chloride 1 L over one hour, with 40 mmol potassium added, plus insulin infusion at rate of four units per hour

Question 8

An 89-year-old woman is admitted following a fall at home. She is found to have a low blood pressure, with readings of 87/54 while lying down and 83/49 on standing. She has a past history of hypertension and ischaemic heart disease; she has not had any regent angina. Her regular medications are aspirin 75 mg od, amlodipine 5 mg od, atorvastatin 20 mg od, bisoprolol 5 mg od, furosemide 40 mg od and lisinopril 5 mg od. She lives alone and mobilises with a two-wheeled frame indoors. On examination, she has moderate bilateral ankle oedema but no other abnormalities are detected. Her initial blood tests are as below:

TABLE 1.2

Investigations.

Haemoglobin	128 g/L (130–180)
White cell count	5.3×10^9/L (4.0–11.0)
Platelet count	246×10^9/L (150–400)
Serum sodium	142 mmol/L (134–145)
Serum potassium	4.4 mmol/L (3.5–4.9)
Serum urea	5.6 mmol/L (2.5–7.0)
Serum creatinine	74 μmol/L (60–110)
Random plasma Glucose	6.7 mmol/L (4.0–7.8)
ECG	Sinus rhythm, rate 71 beats per minute
Chest X-ray	Cardiomegaly

Which of her medications would you discontinue first?

A. amlodipine

B. atorvastatin

C. bisoprolol

D. furosemide

E. lisinopril

Question 9

An 88-year-old woman has been admitted following a non-ST elevation myocardial infarction. Her past medical history includes a stroke, atrial fibrillation and COPD. She lives alone in a bungalow and mobilises with a four-wheeled walking frame indoors only. She has a carer who attends once daily to assist with personal care. What combination of antiplatelet and/or anticoagulant medication would be the most appropriate for her at the time of hospital discharge?

A. apixaban alone

B. apixaban and clopidogrel

C. apixaban, aspirin and clopidogrel

D. apixaban, aspirin, clopidogrel and ticagrelor

E. aspirin, clopidogrel and ticagrelor

Question 10

A 90-year-old man presents with shortness of breath on exertion gradually increasing over several weeks. He does not report any other symptoms, including no change in his bowel motions. He has very little past medical history but has been taking aspirin 75 mg daily for primary cardiovascular prevention for many years. He lives with his wife in a bungalow and is usually independent with self-care.

Blood tests, as below, show that he has a microcytic anaemia that was not present on his last blood test done two years ago.

His aspirin is discontinued, and he is commenced on a proton pump inhibitor drug. After discussing the risks and benefits of endoscopic investigation of his gastrointestinal tract, he decides

TABLE 1.3

Investigations.

Haemoglobin	78 g/L (115–165)
MCV	66 fL (82–100)
White blood cell count	5.3×10^9/L (4.0–11.0)
Platelet count	164×10^9/L (150–400)
Serum ferritin	20 μg/L (15–300)
Serum B$_{12}$	294 ng/L (150–1000)
Serum folate	3.1 μg/L (2.0–11.0)

that he does not want these tests. Which is the best management plan for his anaemia?

A. blood transfusion to haemoglobin >100 g/L
B. check transferrin saturation
C. intravenous iron infusion
D. oral iron tablets once daily
E. oral iron tablets three times daily

Question 11

A 91-year-old woman has been admitted after being found on the floor in her own home by her carers that morning. Her temperature was recorded as 32.3°C when she arrived in the emergency department. Which of the following factors is the most important reason why older people are more susceptible to hypothermia?

A. increased peripheral vasoconstriction
B. lower baseline core body temperature
C. reduced abdominal fat deposition
D. reduced brown adipose tissue metabolism
E. sarcopenia

Question 12

A 79-year-old man is admitted from his care home following a generalised decline over the last five days. He has become less mobile and more confused and agitated than usual. His oral intake has reduced, and he was found on his bedroom floor by the care home staff this morning. On assessment he is hard to rouse and unable to give any verbal history. Physical examination does not show any signs of fluid overload. His blood pressure is 94/57 mmHg, his pulse 95 beats per minute, respiratory rate 16 breaths per minute and his temperature 36.4°C.

Initial blood tests and the most recent prior results are as below:

TABLE 1.4

Investigations.

	Present time	One month ago	
Serum urea	36.1 mmol/L	7.3 mmol/L	(2.5–7.8)
Serum creatinine	298 μmol/L	97 μmol/L	(60–110)

He is commenced on intravenous fluids and his usual medications are initially withheld. What investigation would be most useful at this time?

A. bladder ultrasound scan
B. CT scan of abdomen and pelvis
C. intravenous urography
D. serum autoantibody testing
E. urinalysis for blood and protein

Question 13

A 93-year-old woman of Asian heritage has been admitted to the emergency department, from her care home, complaining of abdominal pain. She describes the pain as constant in nature and localised in her right lower abdomen. The care home staff reported she passed several hundred millilitres of blood in her pad earlier today. Her past history is of hypertension and osteoporosis. She takes ramipril 5 mg daily and alendronate 70 mg weekly. On examination, tenderness is noted in her right lower quadrant with some fullness detected in that area. Her blood pressure is 124/76 mmHg and her pulse 96 beats per minute. An ECG shows her to be in atrial fibrillation. What is the most likely diagnosis?

A. appendicitis

B. colon cancer

C. diverticulitis

D. mesenteric ischaemia

E. ulcerative colitis

Question 14

A 73-year-old man has developed diarrhoea following a course of antibiotics for a suspected urinary tract infection. Stool tests suggest he has developed *Clostridium difficile* associated diarrhoea.

Which of the following criteria is most suggestive of severe disease?

A. abdominal distension and generalised tenderness

B. creatinine 20% above baseline

C. glutamate dehydrogenase (GDH) test positive

D. temperature >37.5°C

E. white cell count >12 × 10⁹/L

Question 15

A 79-year-old woman presents with a one-week history of back pain in the lower thoracic region. Two weeks ago, she was treated with oral trimethoprim for a urinary tract infection by her GP due to dysuria. Her past medical history includes hypertension and type 2 diabetes. Her observations show temperature 37.8°C, blood pressure 146/77 and pulse 85 beats per minute. She is mildly tender in the lower thoracic region, but the rest of the examination is unremarkable.

Her initial investigation results are as below:

TABLE 1.5

Investigations.

Haemoglobin	126 g/L (115–165)
White cell count	12.3 × 10⁹/L (4.0–11.0)
Platelet count	506 × 10⁹/L (150–400)
ESR	78 mm/1st h (<50)
Serum CRP	62 mg/L (<10)

Which action would you take next?

A. request MRI scan of spine

B. request thoracic and lumber spine X-rays

C. send blood cultures

D. send urine for culture

E. start intravenous flucloxacillin

Question 16

A 72-year-old man presents to the emergency department with painful skin lesions. These have been rapidly getting worse over the last two days. On examination he looks unwell with blood pressure 97/62, pulse 118 beats per minute and temperature 38.5°C. There is extensive blistering and epidermal loss over about 20% of his body surface. He also has lesions affecting his oral mucosa. His past medical history is of ischaemic heart disease, COPD and gout. He usually takes aspirin 75 mg od, simvastatin 40 mg at night, allopurinol 200 mg od and a tiotropium inhaler 18 mcg daily. What is the most likely diagnosis?

A. bullous pemphigoid

B. dermatitis herpetiformis

C. exanthematous drug eruption

D. pemphigus vulgaris

E. Stevens-Johnson syndrome

Question 17

A 73-year-old woman with Parkinson's disease is admitted with shortness of breath that started after a brief vomiting illness. It is suspected that she may be developing aspiration pneumonia. Which of the following statements is true of aspiration pneumonia?

A. around 75% of community-acquired pneumonia in older people is thought to be caused by aspiration

B. aspiration while in a supine position is most likely to affect the superior lower-lobe or posterior upper-lobe lung segments

C. detecting aspiration of small volumes during sleep is highly predictive of developing pneumonia

D. most commonly caused by anaerobic organisms

E. typically presents with a lobar pattern

Question 18

A 90-year-old woman is receiving rehabilitation on the orthogeriatric ward following a recent fall and subsequent surgery for fractured neck of femur. She has deteriorated today, and the ward foundation doctor thinks she may have had a pulmonary embolism. Which of the following statements is most likely to be correct regarding pulmonary embolism in older people compared to younger adults?

A. electrocardiogram abnormalities are less common

B. haemoptysis is more common

C. pleuritic chest pain is less common

D. shortness of breath is more common

E. syncope is less common

Question 19

A 77-year-old woman has been admitted to the emergency department with confusion. Her husband reports a period of shaking of all of her limbs lasting around five minutes approximately three hours ago. Since that time, he reports that she has been staring blankly and speaking little. When she does speak, she tends to repeat words or phrases said to her. She is usually independent, but her husband has noticed that her memory has declined recently. She suffered from severe post-natal depression many years ago.

Otherwise, she has little past medical history and takes no regular medications but has a history of penicillin allergy. She does not smoke or drink alcohol. On examination, she is sitting in a chair, and her eyes are open but she is blinking repeatedly. Pupils are equal and normally reactive to light. Tone is normal and she appears to be able to move all four limbs against gravity, but it is difficult to engage her in the examination process. She is unable to accurately answer any questions in a brief cognitive test. The rest of the examination is unremarkable. Her initial blood tests, ECG, chest X-ray and non-contrast CT brain scan did not demonstrate any significant abnormality. Which drug is most likely to be beneficial?

A. aciclovir

B. lorazepam

C. meropenem

D. olanzapine

E. sertraline

Question 20

An 80-year-old man has been admitted following a generalised seizure that was witnessed by the staff of his care home. The seizure is estimated to have lasted around three minutes. Following the seizure, he was confused and disorientated, but this appears to be slowly improving over the few hours since. He has a past history of severe anxiety, ischaemic heart disease and a left partial anterior circulation stroke three years ago. His current medications are clopidogrel 75 mg daily, atorvastatin 40 mg at night and sertraline 50 mg daily. On examination, he has no focal neurological deficits, but mild bradykinesia and a resting tremor are noted in his hands bilaterally. Blood tests, an ECG and a CT brain scan did not show any acute abnormality. It is advised that he be started on an antiepileptic medication due to his risk of recurrent events.

Which drug would you recommend for this man?

A. carbamazepine

B. gabapentin

C. lamotrigine

D. levetiracetam

E. sodium valproate

Question 21

An 80-year-old man with a history of type 2 diabetes has been admitted to hospital following a fall at home. When first seen by the paramedics, his blood glucose was measured as 3.1 mmol/L. Which of the following statements is most accurate regarding hypoglycaemia in older people with type 2 diabetes?

A. dipeptidylpeptidase-4 inhibitors are the diabetes medication class associated with the lowest risk of hypoglycaemia

B. higher risk in people with chronic kidney disease

C. hypoglycaemia results in a similar number of hospital admissions as hyperglycaemia

D. people who live alone are at an increased risk of developing hypoglycaemia

E. sweating and tremor are common warning symptoms

Question 22

A 76-year-old woman, known to have COPD, presents with worsening shortness of breath over the past three days. She has not had any chest pain and is coughing up only small amounts of clear sputum. Examination reveals generalised poor air entry to the chest but no focal signs. Her blood pressure is 134/74, pulse 96 beats per minute, respiratory rate 22 per minute, oxygen saturation 89% on air

and temperature 37.5°C. Her chest X-ray shows hyperexpanded lungs but no consolidation. Her blood gas shows pH 7.36, pO_2 8.7 and pCO_2 5.3. Which of the following is most likely to be beneficial for this woman?

A. aminophylline infusion

B. non-invasive ventilation

C. oral co-amoxiclav

D. oral prednisolone

E. supplemental oxygen to maintain saturations 92%–96%

Question 23

An 80-year-old man develops a painful, swollen left knee while on the ward recovering from pneumonia. Knee joint aspiration is performed, and calcium pyrophosphate crystals are detected along with neutrophils but no organisms. Which of the following blood test abnormalities is associated with the development of this condition?

A. hypernatraemia

B. hypocalcaemia

C. hypomagnesaemia

D. raised alkaline phosphatase

E. thrombocytosis

Question 24

An 80-year-old woman presents to the emergency department complaining of severe abdominal pain, nausea and diarrhoea. Her symptoms started yesterday evening and have become gradually worse. She lives alone, is usually independent, rarely drinks alcohol and is an ex-smoker. Her past medical history includes ischaemic heart disease and a previous stroke. Her current medication is clopidogrel 75 mg once daily, atorvastatin 40 mg at night, bisoprolol 2.5 mg once daily and lisinopril 5 mg once daily. On examination she looks distressed, but her abdomen is soft, bowel sounds are present and she has only mild central abdominal tenderness. Heart sounds are normal, her chest is clear and there is no peripheral oedema. She scores 7 out of 10 on the Abbreviated Mental Test Score. Her ECG shows atrial fibrillation at a rate of 87 beats per minute. Blood tests are normal apart from mildly elevated serum white blood cell count, C-reactive protein and lactate. Which investigation would be most useful?

A. bladder ultrasound scan

B. colonoscopy

C. contrast CT scan abdomen

D. CT angiogram

E. urine culture

Question 25

A 90-year-old woman presented one week ago with severe thoracic back pain, which started following falling over in her own home. An X-ray demonstrated a vertebral fracture at the T10 level. Despite a combination of paracetamol and codeine four times daily, she continues to have severe back pain that limits her functional ability. Which of the following interventions is most likely to help her with her pain control?

A. lidocaine patch

B. percutaneous vertebroplasty

C. soft brace

D. switch codeine to morphine

E. thoracolumbar spinal orthosis

Question 26

A care home has an outbreak of COVID-19. What is the approximate probability of 30-day survival following COVID-19 infection for an unvaccinated person aged over 80 with a Clinical Frailty Score of 6 or 7?

A. 10%

B. 30%

C. 50%

D. 70%

E. 90%

Question 27

A 78-year-old woman is assessed for hypertension in the outpatient clinic. She complains of light-headedness when she stands quickly but has had no recent falls or any history of blackouts. Her blood pressure recorded while lying down was 189/104 mmHg, and one minute after standing was 157/93 mmHg. Her ambulatory blood pressure monitoring shows a daytime average 146/89 mmHg. Which of the following terms best describes this pattern of hypertension?

A. masked hypertension

B. stage 1 hypertension

C. stage 2 hypertension

D. stage 3 hypertension

E. white-coat effect

Question 28

A 75-year-old man presents with an acutely swollen joint. Which of the following factors makes acute calcium pyrophosphate arthritis (pseudogout) more likely than gout?

A. affecting the first tarsometaphalangeal joint

B. hook-like osteophytes seen on X-ray

C. normal serum urate concentration

D. pain maximal within 12 hours of onset

E. redness over the joint

Question 29

Older people are often found to have hyponatraemia at the time of hospital admission. Which drug class is most commonly associated with severe hypo-natraemia (<125 mmol/L) in older people admitted to hospital?

A. antiepileptic drugs

B. loop diuretics

C. proton pump inhibitors

D. serotonin specific reuptake inhibitors

E. thiazide diuretics

Question 30

A 78-year-old woman presents with suspected sepsis. She is usually inde-pendent and lives alone. The critical care team ask what her score is on the quick Sequential (Sepsis-Related) Organ Failure Assessment (qSOFA) score. For which of the following measurements would she score a point on the qSOFA?

A. Glasgow Coma Score 14

B. respiratory rate 18 breaths per minute

C. serum lactate 2.9 mmol/L

D. systolic blood pressure 108 mmHg

E. temperature 38.1°C

Question 31

An 80-year-old woman presents with an acute painful red eye. Which of the following clinical features would be most suggestive of acute angle closure?

A. optic nerve swelling

B. poorly reactive mid-dilated pupil on affected side

C. purulent discharge from the affected eye

D. recent history of eye trauma

E. redness detectable in both eyes

Question 32

An 83-year-old person presents to the emergency department with a painful, red and swollen joint that has developed over the last two days. Regarding septic arthritis in people aged over 80, which of the following is most likely to be correct?

A. a normal serum white blood cell count makes infection unlikely

B. *E. coli* is the most common organism

C. more common in men

D. most people develop pyrexia above 37.5°C

E. the wrist is the joint most commonly affected

Question 33

A 90-year-old woman is admitted following a fall in her care home. She has poor recollection of events. The care home staff found her on the floor in her room with bruising and a small cut around her left temple. Her GCS is 14, but no focal neurological deficit is detected. Which injury is the commonest most significant injury detected on brain CT scans of older people admitted fol-lowing a head injury?

A. extradural haematoma

B. intracerebral bleed or brain contusion

C. skull fracture

D. subarachnoid haemorrhage

E. subdural haematoma

Question 34

An 81-year-old man, born in Cambodia, is admitted from his care home with a his-tory of worsening shortness of breath and a cough productive of sputum. His symp-toms have not responded to two courses of antibiotics in the community. His chest X-ray shows increased shadowing in both upper lungs and hilar lymphadenopathy. Which test would be most useful in estab-lishing if he has active tuberculosis?

A. CT scan of chest, abdomen and pelvis

B. interferon-gamma release assay

C. lymph node biopsy

D. sputum sample for tuberculosis microscopy and culture

E. tuberculin skin test

Question 35

A 74-year-old man presents with a one-week history of nausea, polyuria and drowsiness. He has no past medical history of note. He lives with his wife, is usually independent, occasionally drinks alcohol and is an ex-smoker. Physical examination did not reveal any focal abnormalities, but he scored poorly on a brief cognitive assessment. An ECG and chest X-ray are unremarkable. His blood tests are as shown below.

TABLE 1.6

Investigations.

Serum corrected Calcium	3.26 mmol/L (2.20–2.60)
Plasma parathyroid Hormone (PTH)	1.4 pmol/L (1.6–6.9)
PTH related-protein	0.1 pmol/L (<1.8)
25-hydroxyvitamin D	83 nmol/L (20–100)

Which is the most likely underlying cause of this man's hypercalcaemia?

A. lymphoma

B. multiple myeloma

C. primary hyperparathyroidism

D. prostate cancer

E. squamous cell lung cancer

Question 36

Norovirus is a common cause of acute gastroenteritis in healthcare settings. Which of the following statements is most likely to be correct?

A. a five- to seven-day incubation period is typical

B. after norovirus infection, hospital staff should be 24 hours symptom-free before returning to work

C. alcohol hand-sanitiser gel is similarly effective to handwashing with soap and water

D. spread in healthcare settings is predominantly mediated by contact with contaminated surfaces

E. the duration of symptoms in frail older people is typically three to nine days

Question 37

A 67-year-old man presents with sudden loss of vision to his right eye. He is a type 2 diabetic with evidence of microalbuminuria. He describes his vision as having 'lots of floaters'. Vision in this eye is finger counting only. There is no relative afferent pupillary defect (RAPD) in either eye. You attempt to examine his eye with an ophthalmoscope and notice an absent red reflex in the affected eye. What is your diagnosis for the right eye?

A. cataract

B. diabetic papillopathy

C. exudative diabetic maculopathy

D. rubeosis iridis

E. vitreous haemorrhage

Question 38

A 76-year-old woman with anaemia related to chronic renal failure comes to the acute medical unit complaining of increased tiredness. She is currently using erythropoietin (EPO) injections three times per week and is concerned that she requires an increased dose.

Investigations reveal:

Which of the following is the most appropriate intervention?

A. arrange IV iron supplementation

B. check transferrin saturation

C. do nothing

D. increase the dose of EPO

E. increase the injection frequency of the EPO

TABLE 1.7

Investigations.

Haemoglobin	90 g/L (130–180)
White cell count	6.3 × 10⁹/L (4.0–11.0)
Platelet count	185 × 10⁹/L (130–400)
Serum sodium	136 mmol/L (137–144)
Serum potassium	4.9 mmol/L (3.5–4.9)
Serum creatinine	235 µmol/L (60–110)
Ferritin	7 µg/L (12–200)

Question 39

An 80-year-old woman was admitted with sepsis secondary to pneumonia. She was treated with oxygen, intravenous antibiotics and repeated fluid challenges to a total volume of 4.5 L (equivalent to 60 mL/kg) of sodium chloride 0.9%. On reassessment, her pulse was 132 beats/min, her BP was 72/40 mmHg (mean arterial pressure 54 mmHg [90]) and her respiratory rate was 26 breaths/min. Her oxygen saturation was 92% breathing oxygen 40%. Her central venous pressure was 12 mmHg. In attempting to restore the blood pressure, what is the most appropriate intravenous therapy?

A. colloid

B. dopamine

C. furosemide

D. further crystalloid

E. noradrenaline (norepinephrine)

Question 40

A 78-year-old man with chronic obstructive pulmonary disease presented with a 24-hour history of increased wheeze and breathlessness. He was treated with nebulised salbutamol 2.5 mg and ipratropium 500 micrograms, oral prednisolone 30 mg and oxygen 28% via a Venturi mask. On examination, his pulse was 90 beats per minute and his blood pressure was 146/88 mmHg. His respiratory rate was 26 breaths/min. He had polyphonic wheeze throughout his lung fields.

Investigations:

TABLE 1.8

Investigations.

pO₂	7.3 kPa (11.3–12.6)
pH	7.28 (7.35–7.45)
Bicarbonate	24 mmol/L (21–29)

What is the most appropriate next step in management?

A. bi-level positive airway pressure ventilation

B. increase inspired oxygen to 35%

C. intravenous aminophylline

D. intravenous hydrocortisone

E. reduce inspired oxygen to 24%

Question 41

A 72-year-old woman presented with a one-week history of vomiting and diarrhoea. These symptoms began after she had been to the dentist for a tooth-filling operation. She also complained of feeling dizzy on standing. Her family said that she had been slightly confused and slurred her words.

On examination, her pulse was 114 beats/min and her BP was 85/40 mmHg.

TABLE 1.9

Investigations.

Platelet count	364 × 10⁹/L (150–400)
Serum sodium	123 mmol/L (137–144)
Serum creatinine	123 µmol/L (60–110)

What is the most likely diagnosis?

A. autoimmune adrenal failure (Addison's disease)

B. gastroenteritis

C. hypothyroidism

D. insulinoma

E. syndrome of inappropriate antidiuretic hormone

Question 42

An 83-year-old woman was referred to the acute medical unit for assessment of her palpitations. One hour after arriving, she complained of a return of her palpitations with a central crushing chest pain. She became distressed and agitated. She was given aspirin and sublingual glyceryl trinitrate. On examination, her pulse was very weak and hard to count. Her BP was 88/55 mmHg, her respiratory rate was 20 breaths/min and her oxygen saturation was 98% breathing air. A cardiac monitor was attached and showed a narrow-complex irregular tachycardia with a ventricular rate between 150 and 160 beats per minute. What is the most appropriate next step in management?

A. intravenous adenosine

B. intravenous amiodarone

C. intravenous digoxin

D. intravenous flecainide

E. synchronised cardioversion

Question 43

A 73-year-old man was admitted with a three-day history of progressive leg weakness and poorly localised low back pain. He first noticed tingling and weakness starting in his feet and legs, and then spreading to his upper body and arms. On examination, he had reduced tone in both lower limbs, with grade 4 power of flexion and extension of hips and knees bilaterally, and grade 3 power of foot dorsiflexion and plantar flexion bilaterally. The deep tendon reflexes in his lower limbs were absent, and the plantar responses were flexor. There was loss of all modalities of sensation in both feet in a stocking distribution. Examination of his upper limbs was normal. What respiratory function

variable is it most important to measure regularly?

A. FEV_1

B. forced vital capacity

C. oxygen saturation

D. peak expiratory flow

E. respiratory rate

Question 44

An 89-year-old female presents with distorted vision for two weeks to her right eye only, with straight lines appearing bent. Her left eye has evidence of drusen in the macular area. The fundal picture shows haemorrhage and drusen, visible as yellow lesions adjacent to the haemorrhage.

What would be your likely treatment for this woman?

A. dietary advice

B. intravitreal anti-VEGF therapy

C. laser treatment

D. PDT laser

E. steroid implants

Answers for Chapter 1

1 Correct Answer: A

Explanation: Improved oral hygiene does appear to reduce the risk of aspiration pneumonia, although this has not been proven in nursing home populations. Neither PEG tubes nor thickened fluids have been shown to reduce the risk. All antipsychotic drugs appear to increase the risk of aspiration pneumonia by a similar degree. People living with frailty have a greater risk of aspiration. It is an interesting idea that physical group exercises might reduce the risk, but this has not yet been demonstrated.

Reading

Mandell LA, Niederman MS. Aspiration pneumonia. *N Engl J Med* 2019; 380: 651–663.

2 Correct Answer: B

H—hypertension (uncontrolled)
[1 point]
A—abnormal liver and/or renal function
[1 or 2 points]
S—stroke
[1 point]
B—bleeding tendency
[1 point]
L—labile INR
[1 point]
E—elderly (age >65)
[1 point]
D—drugs (aspirin/NSAIDs) or alcohol excess
[1 point]

A high HAS-BLED score should not be used as a reason not to anticoagulate someone at increased risk of bleeding complications, but instead should be used as a way to help communicate risk and look for potentially reversible factors to improve safety (e.g. control blood pressure, stop aspirin or reduce alcohol intake).

Reading

Lip GYH. Assessing bleeding risk with the HAS-BLED score: Balancing simplicity, practicality, and predictive value in bleeding-risk assessment. *Clin Cardiol* 2015; 38: 562–564.
Pisters R, Lane DA, Nieuwlaat R, et al. A novel user-friendly score (HAS-BLED) to assess 1-year risk of major bleeding in patients with atrial fibrillation: The Euro heart survey. *Chest* 2010; 138: 1093–1100.

3 Correct Answer: B

Explanation: Serum N-terminal pro-B-type natriuretic peptide (NT-proBNP) can be elevated in older age, some other heart diseases, renal impairment (eGFR <60 mL/min/1.73 m^2), sepsis, hypoxia (e.g. pulmonary embolus), chronic obstructive pulmonary disease, diabetes and hepatic cirrhosis. Levels tend to be lower in people of African or African-Caribbean family origin and people with obesity. Treatment with diuretics (including mineralocorticoid antagonists), beta blockers, ACE inhibitors or angiotensin receptor blockers can also cause a reduction. NT-proBNP levels above 2000 ng/L are associated with a worse prognosis and rapid specialist assessment is recommended (within two weeks). An assessment within six weeks is recommended for levels 400–2000 ng/L. Heart failure is unlikely with levels <400 ng/L.

NT-proBNP is sometimes also used in monitoring during treatment for heart failure. Current guidance is to consider measurement as part of a treatment optimisation protocol only in a specialist care setting for people aged under 75 who have heart failure with reduced ejection fraction and an eGFR above 60 mL/min/1.73 m^2 (N.B. average age at the time of heart failure diagnosis in the UK is 77 years).

Reading

National Institute for Health and Care Excellence. Chronic heart failure in adults: Diagnosis and management. Guideline 106, 2018. www.nice.org.uk/guidance/ng106.

4 Correct Answer: C

Explanation: Neuroleptic malignant syndrome is characterised by a combination of hypoactive delirium, increased tone, pyrexia and a history of relevant drug exposure (i.e. prescription of dopamine antagonist or withdrawal of dopamine agonist drugs). There may also be features of autonomic nervous system dysfunction (i.e. raised/fluctuant blood pressure, tachycardia, sweating, nausea and vomiting). Blood tests usually show a raised creatine kinase. It is more common with typical antipsychotics (e.g. haloperidol) but can occur with any antipsychotic drug. The mainstay of treatment is to stop (or restart) the offending drug and supportive care (e.g. hydration). The mortality is around 10%.

Anticholinergic toxicity typically presents with delirium, large pupils, dry mouth and urinary retention. Dementia with Lewy bodies can be associated with neuroleptic drug sensitivity, but it would not explain his pyrexia and tachycardia. The cause of his preadmission decline is likely to be related to his known prior diagnosis of vascular dementia. Serotonin syndrome can cause pyrexia, tachycardia, hypertension, delirium and increased tone. Hyperreflexia and pupillary dilatation would be expected. Sepsis (e.g. UTI) could cause hypoactive delirium, pyrexia and tachycardia, but the increased tone and hypertension are against this.

Reading

Oruch R, Pryme IF, Engelsen BA, et al. Neuroleptic malignant syndrome: An easily overlooked neurologic emergency. *Neuropsychiatr Dis Treat* 2017; 13: 161–175.

5 Correct Answer: D

Explanation: This woman's history suggests that bile salt malabsorption needs to be excluded, e.g. with ^{75}SeHCAT testing. The prior cholecystectomy puts her at increased risk. Microscopic colitis has a macroscopically normal appearance on colonoscopy but abnormal histology obtained from biopsy samples. Some drugs are implicated as potential precipitants— e.g. non-steroidal anti-inflammatory drugs (NSAIDs), proton pump inhibitors (PPIs) and selective serotonin reuptake inhibitors (SSRIs). Treatment is with oral controlled release preparations of budesonide. A faecal calprotectin test can detect bowel inflammation. It is used to help distinguish inflammatory bowel disease from irritable bowel syndrome in people aged <40 but has little use as a diagnostic test in older people. Faecal elastase is used to help detect pancreatic exocrine deficiency. A history of previous pancreatic disease or steatorrhoea would make this a more likely diagnosis. Hydrogen breath tests are sometimes used in the diagnosis of bacterial overgrowth but lack sensitivity or specificity. An empiric trial of antibiotics may be a better approach when this diagnosis is suspected. The risk is increased with diabetes, PPI use, prior intestinal surgery or diverticulosis.

Reading

Arasaradnam RP, Brown S, Forbes A, et al. Guidelines for the investigation of chronic diarrhoea in adults: British Society of Gastroenterology, 3rd edition. *Gut* 2018; 67: 1380–1399.

6 Correct Answer: C

Explanation: Cauda equina syndrome is the diagnosis not to miss here. Around 70% of people have a prior history of chronic back pain, which may insidiously get worse rather than present acutely. Other symptoms can include unilateral or bilateral sciatica, decreased perianal region sensation (may notice while sitting, defaecating or wiping bottom), loss of anal tone, faecal problems (e.g. constipation) and bladder disruption (leading to painless urinary retention with overflow incontinence), lower extremity weakness and reduced sexual function (erectile dysfunction). There may be loss of power, sensation or reflexes in the lower limbs. The key points in the case scenario are back pain, painless urinary retention and reduced leg reflexes. An urgent MRI scan of his spine and then possibly neuro-surgical intervention are required.

Reading

Long B, Koyfman A, Gottlieb M. Evaluation and management of cauda equina syndrome in the emergency department. *Am J Emerg Med* 2020; 38: 143–148.

7 Correct Answer: B

Explanation: The scenario described is hyperosmolar hyperglycaemic syndrome, possibly precipitated by pneumonia and resulting in hypoactive delirium. The key metabolic disturbance is dehydration caused by an osmotic diuresis, which may be made worse by reduced fluid intake (e.g. hypoactive delirium) and any other precipitants (e.g. pneumonia). The aim is to correct the fluid deficit (which could be 8 to 16 L in an 80 kg person) but without causing a too-rapid drop in sodium that could result in central pontine myelinolysis. 0.9% sodium chloride is hypotonic compared to this man's serum and is the fluid of choice. Potassium may be added once his serum glucose falls below 5.5 mmol/L. Fluid correction alone will cause his glucose to fall. An insulin infusion prior to rehydration can cause too rapid a reduction in osmolality or precipitate hypotension.

Reading

Scott AR. Diabetes UK position statement: Management of hyperosmolar hyperglycaemic state in adults with diabetes. *Diabet Med* 2015; 32: 714–724.

8 Correct Answer: A

Explanation: Her ankle oedema is likely to be precipitated, or made worse, by amlodipine. This makes a strong case for discontinuing amlodipine first to help raise her blood pressure and thus reduce the risk of falling. She has not had any recent angina, so this is less of a concern. In the absence of renal impairment, there is not a strong case for stopping lisinopril initially (although in reality it might also be withheld until her blood pressure improves). The furosemide may have been started to help her leg oedema (this is a classic example of a prescription cascade). This drug may not be effective for treating the oedema caused by calcium channel blockers as it is related to vasodilation rather than fluid overload. However, she is not dehydrated and this drug would be expected to have a smaller blood pressure lowering effect. It is possible that it could be stopped later if the oedema resolved on discontinuing amlodipine. She is not bradycardic, and bisoprolol only has a mild effect on blood pressure. Although statin medications can have side effects, including muscle inflammation, there is nothing in the story to suspect this as the cause of her falls. In the longer term it would be necessary, through shared decision-making, to consider the relative risks and benefits of all of her medications as she becomes increasingly frail.

9 Correct Answer: B

Explanation: Following an acute coronary event, ticagrelor is usually recommended in preference to clopidogrel, even for older people, unless bleeding risk is particularly elevated. When the patient is already taking an anticoagulant for atrial fibrillation, adding aspirin seems to increase bleeding risk without any benefit. For the woman in the scenario, with the degree of frailty described, she is at an elevated risk of complications. A reasonable compromise is the combination of clopidogrel with apixaban for a period of six to twelve months.

Reading

Lopes RD, Heizer G, Aronson R, et al. Antithrombotic therapy after acute coronary syndrome or PCI in atrial fibrillation. *N Engl J Med* 2019; 380: 1509–1524.

10 Correct Answer: D

Explanation: Serum ferritin concentrations tend to rise in older age. Values below 15 always indicate iron deficiency, and ones in the range 15 to 44 are probably also iron deficient. A serum transferrin saturation test is usually only helpful in cases of suspected iron overload. Parenteral iron is suitable when oral therapy is not tolerated or not taken reliably or if there is continuing blood loss or malabsorption. In the absence of severe renal disease (including dialysis), there is no evidence that it works more rapidly than oral iron. The scenario does not suggest that any of these apply. Oral iron replacement at lower doses appears to be equally effective and less likely to provoke side effects (e.g. constipation). A blood transfusion does not appear to be indicated at this level of haemoglobin and degree of symptoms.

Reading

Burton JK, Yates LC, Whyte L, et al. New horizons in iron deficiency Anaemia in older adults. *Age Ageing* 2020; 49: 309–318.

Rimon E, Kagansky N, Kagansky M, et al. Are we giving too much iron? Low-dose iron therapy is effective in octogenarians. *Am J Med* 2005; 118: 1142–1147.

11 Correct Answer: E

Explanation: Hypothermia in people aged over 80 is more likely to occur in their own homes and less likely to be associated with alcoholism, self-harm or immersion/drowning incidents than that seen in younger people. Average core body temperature is estimated to be just 0.4°C lower in older people compared to younger people, so only a small factor. Bodily metabolism generates heat and this is in balance with loss from the skin, including evaporation of sweat. Blood flow to the skin is a key mechanism. Vascular dilatation and constriction ability are impaired in older people, making them more susceptible to hypothermia in cold conditions and overheating in hot settings. These changes are probably mediated by reduced sympathetic nervous system activity. Peripheral thermosensor receptors and central brain processing can be impaired in older age. A reduction in vasoconstriction makes hypothermia more likely. Insulating fat prevents heat loss. There is a reduction in the subcutaneous fat layer in old age, but abdominal fat deposition tends to increase. Heat production is proportional to muscle mass, which is reduced by sarcopenia. Reduced activity in general may be a factor, and there may also be attenuation of the shivering response. Brown adipose tissue thermogenesis is thought to be important in newborns but probably not in adults. There may also be behavioural aspects, such as putting on or taking off clothing, which could be affected in cognitive impairment.

Reading

Blatteis CM. Age-dependent changes in temperature regulation: A mini review. *Gerontol* 2012; 58: 289–295.

12 Correct Answer: A

Explanation: This man has an acute kidney injury (classified as stage 3, as his creatinine is more than three times the baseline value). Given the clinical scenario, an obstructed urinary system due to an enlarged prostate and/or constipation is highly likely. A bladder scan would be a quick way to establish if his bladder was full. The other imaging studies suggested would not be appropriate initially. Urinalysis could show evidence of nephritis and autoantibody testing could support a diagnosis of renal pathology, but neither are likely in this scenario.

Reading

NICE guideline. Acute kidney injury: Prevention, detection and management. Published: 18 December 2019. www.nice.org.uk/guidance/ng148.

13 Correct Answer: C

Explanation: Diverticular disease is a cause of intermittent abdominal pain, most commonly in the left lower quadrant. It may be made worse by eating and relieved by passing flatus/stool. There may be constipation, diarrhoea and occasional large rectal bleeds. Diverticular disease is the commonest cause of large lower GI bleeds.

Acute diverticulitis is suggested by constant, severe abdominal pain localising in the left lower quadrant (can be right sided, especially in people of Asian origin) plus fever, change in bowel habit with rectal bleeding/mucus passage or tenderness in the left (or right) lower quadrant and a palpable abdominal mass/distention, often with a previous history of diverticulosis or diverticulitis.

Complications include intra-abdominal abscesses (suggested by a mass on examination or perirectal fullness on digital rectal examination), bowel perforation and peritonitis (abdominal rigidity/guarding on examination), sepsis, fistula into the bladder or vagina (faecaluria, pneumaturia, pyuria or the passage of faeces through the vagina) and intestinal obstruction (colicky abdominal pain, absolute constipation, vomiting or abdominal distention). Abdominal imaging, usually contrast CT, is recommended

for suspected acute complicated diverticulitis with raised inflammatory markers.

Antibiotics are indicated if the person is systemically unwell, is immunosuppressed or has significant comorbidity.

Reading

Diverticular disease: Diagnosis and management. NICE guideline. Published: 27 November 2019. www.nice.org.uk/guidance/ng147.shibl.

Spangler R, Van Pham T, Khoujah D, et al. Abdominal emergencies in the geriatric patient. *Int J Emerg Med* 2014; 7: 43.

14 Correct Answer: A

Explanation: The following suggest severe disease: white blood cell count >15, creatinine 50% above baseline, temperature >38.5°C, or clinical examination or imaging evidence of severe colitis. GDH is a sensitive screening test for the presence of *C. difficile* but lacks the ability to distinguish toxigenic forms.

Reading

Mullish BH, Williams HRT. *Clostridium difficile* infection and antibiotic-associated Diarrhoea. *Clin Med* 2018; 18: 237–241.

15 Correct Answer: C

Explanation: The scenario suggests discitis. The commonest initial complaint is back pain (>90%), and the majority of people have a temperature >37.5°C. CRP >50 and/or ESR >50 are usually present. The risk is increased following an invasive procedure or in those with type 2 diabetes. The causative organism may be identified by blood culture (around two thirds of cases), but tissue biopsy/aspiration of collection (e.g. CT-guided) may be required (chances of finding the organism better if not on antibiotics). It can be caused by a range of possible organisms, so finding the cause is important.

The commonest causative organism is *Staphylococcus aureus* (including MRSA) (around 40%), but other organisms include *Escherichia coli* or Group B β-haemolytic streptococcus. Sometimes the organism remains unidentified (around 25%). Discitis is usually detected by MRI scanning but can sometimes be visualised on CT scans. Antibiotic treatment is initially intravenous (at least one week) with a total duration of at least six weeks.

Reading

Hopkinson N, Patel K. Clinical features of septic discitis in the UK: A retrospective case ascertainment study and review of management recommendations. *Rheumatol Int* 2016; 36: 1319–1326.

16 Correct Answer: E

Explanation: Stevens-Johnson syndrome and toxic epidermal necrolysis (TEN) are related conditions and represent the most severe forms of cutaneous drug reaction. They are characterised by extensive epidermal loss with mucous membrane erosions. The lesions are painful with blistering. Patients are pyrexial and systemically unwell. In TEN, a greater proportion of the body is affected by these lesions (>30%) and the prognosis is worse (mortality >40%). Potential causative drugs include antibacterial sulfonamides, anticonvulsants, oxicam-NSAIDs and allopurinol. It usually occurs within four days to four weeks of drug commencement but can be triggered by other stimuli, including infections and radiotherapy.

Reading

Marzano AV, Borghi A, Cugno M. Adverse drug reactions and organ damage: The skin. *Eur J Intern Med* 2016; 28: 17–24.

17 Correct Answer: B

Explanation: It is estimated that 5% to 15% of community-acquired pneumonia is due to aspiration (but this figure is likely be a little higher in older people with frailty). Chest imaging findings include infiltrates in the gravity-dependent lung segments if the patient is supine when the aspiration occurs (i.e. superior lower-lobe or posterior upper-lobe segments). Micro-aspiration of small volumes of the oropharyngeal contents during sleep is surprisingly common even among healthy people and does not usually suggest pneumonia is imminent. Studies suggest that aerobic organisms cause most of the pneumonias following aspiration. Anaerobic organisms may only be important when lung abscesses develop. A bronchopneumonia pattern is more common than a lobar one.

Reading

Mandell LA, Niederman MS. Aspiration pneumonia. *N Engl J Med* 2019; 380: 651–663.

18 Correct Answer: C

Explanation: Comparing older people with pulmonary embolism to younger people, dyspnoea occurs at a similar frequency (about 80%) but pleuritic chest pain is less common in the old (about 50% vs 75%). Fewer older people have haemoptysis (about 8% vs 25%), and more present with syncope. ECG changes in pulmonary embolus are typically non-specific and tend to be present only in more severe cases. There's no reason to think they are less likely to occur in older people.

Reading

Kokturk N, Oguzulgen IK, Demir N, et al. Differences in clinical presentation of pulmonary embolism in older vs younger patients. *Circ J* 2005; 69: 981–986.

Stein PD, Gottschalk A, Saltzman HA, et al. Diagnosis
   of acute pulmonary embolism in the elderly. *J Am
   Coll Cardiol* 1991; 18: 1452–1457.

19 Correct Answer: B

Explanation: Non-convulsive   status
epilepticus is suggested by the seizure at onset of her symptoms, echo-
lalia (repetition) and automatisms
(e.g. repetitive blinking). The history
of memory decline could suggest the
development of underlying neurodegenerative pathology, increasing her
risk of seizures. An electroencephalo-
gram would be the key investigation
ideally, if not always actually performed in clinical practice. The seizure
activity might be terminated by intravenous lorazepam.

Reading

Woodford HJ, George J, Jackson M. Non-convulsive
   status epilepticus: A practical approach to diagnosis
   in confused older people. *Postgrad Med J* 2015; 91:
   655–661.

20 Correct Answer: C

Explanation: Epilepsy in older people
is usually focal at onset, which may be
followed by secondary generalisation.
Often there is underlying pathology,
including cerebrovascular disease, neurodegenerative disease or brain tumours.
Efficacy in seizure control appears to
be similar between the different available antiepileptic drugs. Carbamazepine
is usually less well tolerated. The 2018
SIGN guidance recommends lamotrigine
or levetiracetam for focal-onset seizures
in older people. Sodium valproate can
cause Parkinsonism, which suggests it is
not ideal for this man. Levetiracetam can
cause anxiety, so might also be avoided
here.

Reading

Scottish Intercollegiate Guidelines Network. Diagnosis
   and management of epilepsy in adults. Guideline
   143, 2018.
Sen A, Jette N, Husain M, et al. Epilepsy in older people. *Lancet* 2020; 395: 735–748.

21 Correct Answer: B

Explanation: Metformin is the medication with lowest risk of hypoglycaemia;
insulin has the highest risk. Chronic
kidney disease, cardiovascular disease,
dementia, frailty and alcohol use all
increase the risk. Living alone probably does not. Hypoglycaemia is a more
common reason for hospital admission
than hyperglycaemia, especially among
older people with diabetes. Sympathetic
system-mediated symptoms (e.g. sweating, palpitations and tremor) become
less common in older people, and more
people present with symptoms caused by
reduced brain glucose (e.g. confusion,
slurred speech or visual disturbances).

Reading

Freeman J. Management of hypoglycemia in older
   adults with type 2 diabetes. *Postgrad Med* 2019;
   131: 241–250.
Lipska KJ, Ross JS, Wang Y, et al. National trends
   in US hospital admissions for hyperglycemia and
   hypoglycemia among Medicare beneficiaries, 1999
   to 2011. *JAMA Intern Med* 2014; 174: 1116–1124.

22 Correct Answer: D

Explanation: During exacerbations of
COPD, short-acting beta-2 agonists (+/-
short-acting antimuscarinics) are the
bronchodilators of choice. Nebulisers
may be easier to administer while
acutely unwell but are probably no more
effective than correctly used inhalers.
Theophylline/aminophylline are no longer recommended due to side effects.
Oral prednisolone is typically given for

five days. Exacerbations can be triggered by a variety of stimuli, including viral infections, and antibiotics are not always required. Increased cough and sputum purulence are signs that antibiotics may be beneficial. Supplemental oxygen may be required to maintain saturations in the target range of 88%–92%. Blood gas testing is used to detect rising carbon dioxide or worsening acidosis, which can be indications for non-invasive ventilation.

Reading

Global strategy for the diagnosis, management, and prevention of chronic obstructive pulmonary disease. GOLD 2020. www.goldcopd.org.

23 Correct Answer: C

Explanation: The description is of acute calcium pyrophosphate crystal arthritis (pseudogout). This most commonly affects the knee, with the wrist next most likely to be affected. It is rare in younger people. Acute attacks can be triggered by other illnesses, trauma or operations. It can also occur secondary to a number of disorders, including hyperparathyroidism, haemochromatosis and hypomagnesaemia. X-rays may detect chondrocalcinosis (a line of calcium along the articular cartilage).

Reading

Rosenthal AK, Ryan LM. Calcium pyrophosphate deposition disease. *N Engl J Med* 2016; 374: 2575–2584.

24 Correct Answer: D

Explanation: Mesenteric ischaemia is the commonest form of acute bowel ischaemia. It should be suspected if the degree of abdominal pain is out of keeping with abdominal signs (i.e. more severe than

expected due to the visceral, rather than peritoneal, origin of pain). Nausea, vomiting and diarrhoea may also be present. Superior mesenteric artery embolus is the most common form, usually from a cardiac source (e.g. atrial fibrillation). It can be detected by CT angiography. Serum lactate elevation may only be a late feature. The mortality rate is over 50% in older people.

Reading

Spangler R, Van Pham T, Khoujah D, et al. Abdominal emergencies in the geriatric patient. *Int J Emerg Med* 2014; 7: 43.

25 Correct Answer: D

Explanation: There is no evidence to support the efficacy of lidocaine patches for management of pain due to bone fracture. Vertebroplasty has little evidence of efficacy for pain control. Also, neither soft nor rigid braces (e.g. thoracolumbar spinal orthosis) appear to be effective. Adequate analgesia (e.g. escalation to a stronger opioid drug) is most likely to help, along with physiotherapy.

Reading

Goodwin VA, Hall AJ, Rogers E, et al. Orthotics and taping in the management of vertebral fractures in people with osteoporosis: A systematic review. *BMJ Open* 2016; 6: e010657.

Percutaneous vertebroplasty and percutaneous balloon kyphoplasty for treating osteoporotic vertebral compression fractures. Technology appraisal guidance 2013. nice.org.uk/guidance/ta279

Williams H, Carlton E. Topical lignocaine patches in traumatic rib fractures. *Emerg Medicine J* 2015; 32: 333–334.

26 Correct Answer: D

Explanation: A mortality rate of 34% has been reported among care home residents with a median age of 83.

Reading

McMichael TM, Currie DW, Clark S, et al. Epidemiology of Covid-19 in a long-term care facility in King County, Washington. *N Engl J Med* 2020; 382: 2005–2011.

27 Correct Answer: B

Explanation: This pattern best matches stage 1 hypertension. The higher BP while lying should be overlooked, in favour of the standing BP value, when a significant postural drop or symptoms suggesting orthostatic hypotension are present.

Masked hypertension: blood pressure readings taken in the clinic are within the accepted normal range but are then higher on average daytime ambulatory blood pressure monitoring or average home blood pressure values.

Stage 1 hypertension: clinic blood pressure recordings 140/90 mmHg to 159/99 mmHg and daytime ambulatory/home averages 135/85 mmHg to 149/94 mmHg.

Stage 2 hypertension: clinic blood pressure recordings 160/100 mmHg to 179/119 mmHg and daytime ambulatory/home averages 150/95 mmHg or higher.

Stage 3 or severe hypertension: clinic systolic blood pressure 180 mmHg or higher or clinic diastolic blood pressure 120 mmHg or higher.

White-coat effect: daytime ambulatory/home blood pressure averages more than 20/10 mmHg lower than clinic values.

Reading

National Institute for Health and Care Excellence. Hypertension in adults: Diagnosis and management. Guideline 136, 2019. www.nice.org.uk/guidance/ng136.

28 Correct Answer: B

Explanation: Acute gout, calcium pyrophosphate (CPP, 'pseudogout') and septic arthritis can usually not be distinguished by clinical examination and blood tests, and they may co-exist within a joint. Examination of the synovial fluid is required. Gout is suggested by severe pain reaching its maximum within 6 to 12 hours of onset, with erythema and tenderness around joint. Gout is also more likely when it affects the first tarsometaphalangeal joint or when tophi are detected. Attacks tend to last between a few days and a week. Risk factors include male gender, hypertension, obesity, cardiovascular disease, chronic renal failure, use of diuretics, a diet high in purine-rich foods and alcohol consumption. Serum urate concentrations cannot confirm or exclude gout (it can be high in people without gout and normal in people with acute gout).

Calcium pyrophosphate deposition disease is the modern term for pseudogout. It may occur secondary to a number of disorders, including hyperparathyroidism, haemochromatosis and hypomagnesaemia. X-rays may reveal chondrocalcinosis (a line of calcium along the articular cartilage) or hook-like osteophytes. Acute CPP disease causes mono- or oligo-articular arthritis. It is rare below the age of 60. Affected joints are hot, red and swollen—it can be hard to distinguish from acute gout and septic arthritis. The knee is affected most commonly, then the wrist. The first metatarsophalangeal joint is rarely affected. There may be associated pyrexia. Acute attacks can be provoked by other acute illnesses or trauma (e.g. following hip fracture). Attacks can last several weeks. Chronic CPP disease can cause a clinical picture similar to osteoarthritis.

Acute attacks of either condition can be treated with steroids (oral or intra-articular), colchicine or NSAIDs. All of these are potentially harmful to older patients. In the longer term, the prevention of recurrence of gout is achieved by using urate-lowering therapy (e.g. allopurinol) and dietary modification.

Reading

Ma L, Cranney A, Holroyd-Leduc JM. Acute mono-arthritis: What is the cause of my patient's painful swollen joint? *CMAJ* 2009; 180: 59–65.

Rosenthal AK, Ryan LM. Calcium pyrophosphate deposition disease. *N Engl J Med* 2016; 374: 2575–2584.

29 Correct Answer: B

Explanation: A study found that loop diuretics were taken by 71% of older people (mean age 84) admitted to hospital with severe hyponatraemia. 66% were taking PPIs, 21% thiazide diuretics, 3% SSRIs and 1% carbamazepine.

Reading

Zhang X, Li X. Prevalence of hyponatremia among older in-patients in a general hospital. *Eur Geriatr Med* 2020. 11(4): 685–692. doi: 10.1007/s41999-020-00320-3.

30 Correct Answer: A

Explanation: The quick Sequential (Sepsis-Related) Organ Failure Assessment (qSOFA) score assigns one point for systolic hypotension (≤100 mmHg), tachypnoea (≥22/min) or altered mentation (defined as anything other than GCS 15), giving a total score between zero and three.

Reading

Seymour CW, Liu VX, Iwashyna TJ, et al. Assessment of clinical criteria for sepsis for the third international consensus definitions for sepsis and septic shock (Sepsis-3). *JAMA* 2016; 315: 762–774.

31 Correct Answer: B

Explanation: Acute angle closure is suggested by a unilateral onset of a red, swollen eye with a dull pain in that area. Vision is usually blurred with haloes around lights. There is reduced visual acuity, corneal oedema, a fixed or poorly reactive mid-dilated pupil and elevated intraocular pressure. A bilateral presentation, absence of pain, purulent discharge, optic nerve swelling, a history of recent trauma and normal pupil reactions are against the diagnosis. The term 'glaucoma' is reserved for people with confirmed optic neuropathy.

Reading

Flores-Sanchez BC, Tatham AJ. Acute angle closure glaucoma. *Br J Hosp Med* 2019; 80: C174–C179.

32 Correct Answer: D

Explanation: Knee and shoulder are the joints most often affected by septic arthritis. Around a quarter of infections in the over 80s occur in prosthetic joints, and around 10% of cases have more than one joint affected. Around half of patients have normal serum white cell count but almost all have elevations in ESR and/or CRP. Around 30% have temperatures below 37.8°C at presentation. The most common causative organisms are staphylococcus or streptococcus species. Infections with organisms such as *E. coli* and pseudomonas are possible. The mortality rate is around 10% aged over 80. Septic arthritis is more common in women after age 80, whereas it is more common in men in younger age groups.

Reading

Gavet F, Tournadre A, Soubrier M, et al. Septic arthritis in patients aged 80 and older: A comparison with younger adults. *J Am Geriatr Soc* 2005; 53: 1210–1213.

33 Correct Answer: E

Explanation: The frequency of injury deemed the most significant was reported in a UK case series: subdural haematoma 45%, soft tissue injury or skull fracture 21%, subarachnoid haemorrhage 19%, cerebral contusion or intracerebral haemorrhage 14% and extradural haematoma 2%.

Reading

Hawley C, Sakr M, Scapinello S, et al. Traumatic brain injuries in older adults—6 years of data for one UK trauma centre: Retrospective analysis of prospectively collected data. *Emerg Med J* 2017; 34: 509–516.

34 Correct Answer: D

Explanation: Around 30% of TB deaths worldwide occur in people aged 65 and over. At presentation the prevalence of cough, sputum, weight loss and fatigue/malaise are similar to that of younger people, but fever (>38°C), sweating and haemoptysis occur less frequently.

Latent tuberculosis (TB) infection can become active again in older people. A 5%–10% lifetime risk of progressing to active TB has been estimated. Immunodeficiency states such as HIV infection, immunosuppression (e.g. organ transplantation or rheumatoid arthritis), smoking, diabetes and severe chronic renal impairment increase the risk.

Tuberculin skin testing (also called the Mantoux test) involves an intradermal injection and is used to identify latent TB. The response wanes with immunosenescence and has around a 30% false negative rate overall and with a decline in sensitivity in old age (<10% beyond age 90) and a few false positive results. It can also be affected by the use of immunosuppressant medications. Interferongamma release assay is a blood test that may be more sensitive for detecting latent TB.

Regarding the diagnosis of active TB, sputum samples (when obtainable) seem to perform similarly for diagnosis as in younger people. Lymph node biopsy is an option, especially for non-pulmonary TB. Adverse effects of treatment (e.g. hepatotoxicity with isoniazid, rifampicin and pyrazinamide; ocular toxicity with ethambutol) are more common in older people, and treatment success rates are lower.

Reading

Khan A, Rebhan A, Seminara D, et al. Enduring challenge of latent tuberculosis in older nursing home residents: A brief review. *J Clin Med Res* 2019; 11: 385–390.

National Institute for Health and Care Excellence. Tuberculosis. NICE Guideline 33, 2016. www.nice. org.uk/guidance/ng33.

Yew WW, Yoshiyama T, Leung CC, et al. Epidemiological, clinical and mechanistic perspectives of tuberculosis in older people. *Respirology* 2018; 23: 567–575.

35 Correct Answer: B

Explanation: Hypercalcaemia can cause polyuria, nausea, vomiting and constipation, which can lead to dehydration. Cognitive impairment, anxiety and depression may also occur. Renal calculi, pancreatitis and peptic ulceration (related to increased gastrin secretion) are possible. Most cases are due to either primary hyperparathyroidism or hypercalcaemia of malignancy. An elevated PTH suggests primary hyperparathyroidism. This is often detected by chance in asymptomatic individuals with longstanding small increases in calcium. Parathyroid cancer is a rare possibility (very high PTH). Hypercalcaemia of malignancy is more likely to present as an emergency with marked symptoms and is a poor prognostic sign. Humoral hypercalcemia of malignancy (i.e. elevated PTH-related protein [PTHrP]) is the commonest form of cancer-related hypercalcaemia (80%), most commonly due to underlying squamous cell cancer (lung, head and neck, oesophagus, skin or cervix) or breast, kidney, prostate or bladder cancers. Bone osteolysis is another possibility, which is caused by tumour secretion of osteoclast-activating cytokines most commonly seen in patients with breast cancer or multiple myeloma (20% of cancer-related hypercalcaemia). In this situation the PTHrP level will not be elevated. A rare cause is excess vitamin D production by lymphomas (<1%).

Reading

Zagzag J, Hu MI, Fisher SB, et al. Hypercalcemia and cancer: Differential diagnosis and treatment. *CA Cancer J Clin* 2018; 68: 377–386.

36 Correct Answer: E

Explanation: Noroviruses are non-enveloped RNA viruses and are a common cause of acute gastroenteritis. There is a 12- to 48-hour incubation period followed by abdominal cramps, watery diarrhoea, nausea and vomiting. Some people, however, may have vomiting or diarrhoea alone and some are asymptomatic (maybe a third of infections). Associated systemic symptoms can occur (e.g. myalgia, low-grade fever). The duration is two to three days in non-frail people, but in frail older people symptoms may last three to nine days. Older people are more likely to be hospitalised, develop complications (e.g. aspiration pneumonia) and die.

Norovirus is highly contagious due to high viral shedding in faeces and vomitus, low infectious dose required and environmental stability of the organism. 75% of cases occur in cooler months. Viral evolution prevents the development of immunity. Outbreaks are particularly common in hospitals and care homes.

Person-to-person contact accounts for the majority of transmission in healthcare settings. Stool samples are the usual way to diagnose infection, but rectal swabs and vomitus testing are possible.

The virus can still be shed in stools once diarrhoea has resolved. Contact with others should be avoided and staff should be excluded until 48 hours symptom-free. Environmental cleaning and chemical disinfection are essential to interrupt the chain of virus transmission. Handwashing with soap and water is the preferred method to prevent infection. The efficacy of alcohol hand gel against noroviruses is controversial and efficacy is uncertain. The additional use of gown and gloves is recommended.

Reading

Cardemil CV, Parashar UD, Hall AJ. Norovirus infection in older adults: Epidemiology, risk factors, and opportunities for prevention and control. *Infect Dis Clin North Am* 2017; 31: 839–870.

Chen Y, Hall AJ, Kirk MD. Norovirus disease in older adults living in long-term care facilities: Strategies for management. *Curr Geriatr Rep* 2017; 6: 26–33.

37 Correct Answer: E

Explanation: Vitreous haemorrhage is likely to be caused by neovascularisation due to proliferative diabetic retinopathy (PDR). There is an increased risk of PDR in patients with renal impairment and type 1 diabetes mellitus. Cataract visual loss is gradual as opposed to sudden in this case. Also, floaters are not consistent with cataracts. Visual loss in diabetic papillopathy is also gradual; a RAPD will be present along with a normal red reflex. Floaters and absent red reflex are not consistent with maculopathy.

38 Correct Answer: A

Explanation: Iron replacement is the most important step in patients with chronic kidney disease where the ferritin is below 100. Although the patient is requesting a change in EPO dose, it is not appropriate given that the ferritin is below target (65 vs target level of >100). As such, the optimal next step is iron supplementation. If the haemoglobin fails to recover despite ferritin >100, then a change in EPO dose can be considered.

Reading

NICE Pathways. Anaemia of chronic kidney disease: ESA therapy. https://pathways.nice.org.uk/pathways/anaemia-management-in-people-with-chronic-kidney-disease.

39 Correct Answer: E

Explanation: As vascular tone depression is a hallmark of septic shock, administration of noradrenaline (norepinephrine) is logical in this setting.

Reading

NICE guidance 'Sepsis: Recognition, diagnosis and early management' 2017. www.nice.org.uk/guidance/ng51.

Scheeren TWL, et al. Current use of vasopressors in septic shock. *Ann Intensive Care* 2019; 9 (1): 20.

40 Correct Answer: A

Explanation: This question describes worsening type 2 respiratory failure in a patient with chronic obstructive pulmonary disease. Arterial blood gas measurement is needed prior to and following starting non-invasive ventilation (NIV). For most patients with an acute exacerbation of COPD, the initial management should be optimal medical therapy and targeting oxygen saturation 88%–92%. NIV should be started when pH <7.35 and pCO_2 >6.5 kPa persist or develop despite optimal medical therapy.

Reading

British Thoracic Society/Intensive Care Society guidelines. Ventilatory management of acute hypercapnic respiratory failure in adults. 2016.

41 Correct Answer: A

Explanation: Typical history of gastrointestinal upset, with low sodium, high potassium and low glucose. Symptoms triggered by an operation, dental or medical procedure such as a tooth filling can occur in Addison's disease.

Reading

Addison's disease. www.nhs.uk/conditions/addisons-disease/treatment/.

42 Correct Answer: E

Explanation: This question relates to the Resuscitation Council's (UK) 'Advanced Life Support Guidelines' (2015), which can be tested in the Specialty Certificate Examination. Unstable patients with supraventricular tachycardia and a pulse are treated with synchronised cardioversion.

Reading

Resuscitation Council UK. Resuscitation guidelines, 2015. www.resus.org.uk/library/2015-resuscitation-guidelines.

43 Correct Answer: B

Explanation: This question describes a typical case of Guillain-Barré syndrome (acute idiopathic demyelinating polyneuropathy). The best test of respiratory muscle function in this case is forced vital capacity (FVC). FVC is the maximum volume of air expired from the lungs after a maximum inspiration, and it should be monitored in patients with neuromuscular weakness. FVC is a simple, widely available measure of the strength of respiratory muscles. As the validity of FVC is dependent on technique, the best of three readings should be recorded.

44 Correct Answer: B

Explanation: Lesions on the macular include drusen, pigmentation or atrophy. If there is any haemorrhage, then conversion to wet age-related macular degeneration (ARMD) is strongly suspected. This patient needs to be referred to the hospital eye clinic service. NICE approved treatment for this condition, providing the vision is within the criteria, is monthly intravitreal anti-vascular endothelial growth factor (VEGF) therapy. Haemorrhage is not consistent with diabetic-related eye disease. There is no evidence of diabetic retinopathy in the affected eye, and there are no changes in the opposing eye. Dry macular changes would only consist of the drusen; there would be no evidence of macular oedema or haemorrhage. Photodynamic therapy (PDT) laser was the treatment for wet ARMD pre-anti-VEGF.

Reading

Patient information leaflet. Anti-VEGF intravitreal injection treatment, Moorfields Eye Hospital NHS Foundation Trust. www.moorfields.nhs.uk/sites/default/files/uploads/documents/Patient%20information%20-%20intravitreal%20injections%20for%20AMD.pdf.

2

Basic Science and Gerontology

LEARNING OBJECTIVE:

An ability to understanding the basic science and biology of ageing, and being able to give advice on, and promote, healthy ageing.

- Recognition that good health includes both physical and mental wellbeing and social, sexual and spiritual aspects.
- Factors influencing health status in older people.
- The biology of healthy ageing in humans, including in relation to changes in fluid and electrolyte homeostasis, thermoregulation and hypothalamic-pituitary axis.
- The effect of ageing on the different organ systems (including skin, urogenitary and digestive tract) and homeostasis.
- The effect of ageing on functional ability.
- Pathophysiology of frailty and sarcopenia.
- Main demographic trends in UK society.
- The basic elements of the psychology of ageing.
- Clinical pharmacology and therapeutics for older people.
- Pathophysiology of pain.
- Ageism and strategies to counteract this.
- Healthy ageing across the life course and prevention of disability and illness.

- The nature of research in older adults and the application of this to individuals.

Questions

Question 45

Which of the following statements is true regarding classical Hutchinson-Gilford progeria syndrome (HGPS)?

A. cancer risk is high, including thyroid neoplasms, melanoma, meningioma, soft tissue sarcomas, hematologic/lymphoid cancers and osteosarcomas

B. causative gene is WRN

C. inheritance is autosomal dominant

D. main symptoms include a lack of the pubertal growth spurt during early teen years, greying or loss of hair, scleroderma-like skin lesions and characteristic facies

E. onset of symptoms is usually second to third decade of life (adulthood progeria)

Question 46

Which of the following statements concerning the ageing of skin is true?

A. acute inflammation is recognised as a major cause of skin ageing
B. gene mutations are not thought to be associated with distinct ageing syndromes
C. no class of wavelength of light has found to increase DNA damage in the skin
D. reactive oxygen species play a critical rôle in dermal extracellular matrix alterations of both intrinsic ageing and photoageing
E. telomeres become longer with each cell division and ultimately result in cellular senescence and limited numbers of cell division

Question 47

Which one of these drugs used in older patients is typically involved with phase II metabolism?

A. amitryptiline
B. diazepam
C. ibuprofen
D. phenytoin
E. procainamide

Question 48

Which of the following statements is true concerning the health status of older people?

A. addressing inequalities would be expected to have little effect on the burden of ill health
B. as people age, they become less susceptible to disability
C. 'compression of morbidity' theory suggests that it would be beneficial to bring to a younger age the onset of chronic illness
D. having fewer symptoms is associated with a higher quality of life
E. improving education and financial opportunities would be expected to have little effect on the health of older adults

Question 49

Which of the following statements is true about current UK demographic trends?

A. by 2032, 11.3 million people are expected to be living on their own, more than 40% of all households
B. men and women in the highest socio-economic class can, on average, expect to live about as long as those in the lowest socio-economic class, but more of those years will be disability-free
C. the number of deaths each year is expected to decrease by about 15%
D. over time, birth rates have remained relatively stable
E. over the 20 years from 2012 to 2032, the population in England is predicted to decrease by eight million

Question 50

Concerning exercise in older age, which of the following statements is correct?

A. allowing people with dementia to wander reduces the risk of developing delirium
B. people at risk of falls should mobilise less frequently
C. randomised controlled studies have shown that exercise reduces the risk of developing dementia
D. the risks of exercise outweigh the benefits in older people with moderate to severe frailty
E. weight training is inappropriate for people living with frailty

Question 51

Which of the following statements regarding smoking and alcohol is most likely to be true for older people?

A. in severe frailty there is no benefit in stopping smoking and this simply deprives people of a comfort

B. older people are more likely to binge drink alcohol than younger people are

C. regular drinkers have lower rates of depression

D. regular moderate alcohol consumption is associated with a lower risk of developing dementia

E. the increased risk of dementia in smokers is not reversed by stopping smoking

Question 52

With respect to oral health and fluid intake, which of the following statements is most likely to be correct for older people?

A. around 60% of people in care homes are dehydrated

B. dentures should be worn overnight to prevent gum atrophy

C. people with dementia have lower rates of dental problems

D. poor dental health increases the risk of aspiration pneumonia

E. the presence of urinary incontinence has no impact on a person's fluid intake

Question 53

Which model of ageing is frequently associated with the infiltration of immune cells as well as the release of pro-inflammatory cytokines such as interleukin 6 (IL-6) and interleukin 8 (IL-8)?

A. cellular senescence

B. chronic 'sterile' inflammation

C. macromolecular dysfunction

D. progenitor cell function decline

E. somatic inevitability

Answers for Chapter 2

45 Correct Answer: C

The two commonest progeria syndromes can be compared as follows:

TABLE 2.1

Comparison of HGPS and Werner syndrome.

	HGPS	Werner syndrome
Causative gene	LMNA (de novo dominant mutation)	WRN (autosomal recessive mutations)
Inheritance	Autosomal dominant (de novo)	Autosomal recessive
Onset of symptoms	First year of life (childhood progeria)	Second to third decade of life (adulthood progeria)
Main symptoms	Severe failure to thrive in infancy. Progressive alopecia leading to total alopecia. Skin lesions. Characteristic facies. Loss of subcutaneous fat. Bone changes. Skeletal anomalies. Musculoskeletal degeneration. Hearing loss.	Lack of the pubertal growth spurt during early teen years. Greying or loss of hair. Scleroderma-like skin lesions. Characteristic facies.

(Continued)

TABLE 2.1

Comparison of HGPS and Werner syndrome. (Continued)

	HGPS	Werner syndrome
Cancer risk	Not reported	High risk of cancer, including thyroid neoplasms, melanoma, meningioma, soft tissue sarcomas, hematological/lymphoid cancers and osteosarcomas

Reading

Conn's Handbook of Models for Human Aging. Chapter 2, Premature Aging Syndrome, Fabio Coppedè (University of Pisa, Pisa, Italy).

46 Correct Answer: D

Explanation: Reactive oxygen species play a critical rôle in dermal extracellular matrix alterations of both intrinsic ageing and photoageing.

Persistently exposing skin to ultra-violet radiation increases DNA damage and mutations and leads to premature ageing or carcinogenesis. Telomeres are repetitive nucleotide sequences which become shorter with each cell division and ultimately result in cellular senescence and limited numbers of cell division. Gene mutation is inherited and causes progeria, a type of premature ageing, often showing accelerated skin ageing phenotype, including skin atrophy and sclerosis, poikiloderma, alopecia, thinning and greying of the hair. Chronic, low-grade inflammation is also recognised as a major characteristic of the ageing process. This phenomenon is called 'inflammageing.'

Reading

Zhang S, Duan E. Fighting against skin aging: The way from bench to bedside. *Cell Transplant* 2018; 27 (5): 729–738.

47 Correct Answer: E

Procainamide. The others are typically associated with phase I metabolism.

Reading

Hutchison LC, O'Brien CE. Changes in pharmacokinetics and pharmacodynamics in the elderly patient. *J Pharm Pract* 2007; 20: 4–12.

48 Correct Answer: D

A higher symptom burden is a factor related to a lower health-related quality of life.

Reducing socio-economic disparities in health by improving the access to education and by providing financial opportunities should be among the priorities in improving the health of older adults. As people age, they become more susceptible to disease and disability. Much of the burden of ill health among older people can be reduced or prevented by adequately addressing specific risk factors, including injury, development of noncommunicable diseases, poverty, social isolation and exclusion, mental health disorders and elder maltreatment.

'Compression of morbidity' theory states,

most illness was chronic and occurred in later life and postulated that the lifetime burden of illness could be reduced if the onset of chronic illness could be postponed and if this postponement could be greater than increases in life expectancy.

(Fries, 2003)

Reading

Fries JF. Measuring and monitoring success in compressing morbidity. *Ann Intern Med* 2003; 139 (5 Pt 2): 455–459.

Jagger C, Matthews FE, Wohland P, et al. A comparison of health expectancies over two decades in England: Results of the cognitive function and ageing study I and II. *Lancet* 2016; 387: 779–786.

Klompstra L, Ekdahl AW, Krevers B, Milberg A, Eckerblad J. Factors related to health-related quality of life in older people with multimorbidity and high health care consumption over a two-year period. *BMC Geriatr* 2019; 19 (1): 187.

Kollia N, Caballero FF, Sánchez-Niubó A, et al. Social determinants, health status and 10-year mortality among 10,906 older adults from the English longitudinal study of aging: The ATHLOS project. *BMC Public Health* 2018; 18 (1): 1357.

Risk factors of ill health among older people. www.euro.who.int/en/health-topics/Life-stages/healthy-ageing/data-and-statistics/risk-factors-of-ill-health-among-older-people.

49 Correct Answer: A

Prediction of demographic trends could form the basis of an SBA question, and it is therefore important for you to have an approximate idea of the figures involved. By 2032, 11.3 million people are expected to be living on their own—more than 40% of all households. The number of people over 85 living on their own is expected to grow from 573,000 to 1.4 million. Over time, birth rates have fluctuated quite significantly. Current predictions are that the annual number of births will level off to around 680,000–730,000 births per year. The number of deaths each year is expected to grow by 13% from 462,000 to 520,000 by 2032. Men and women in the highest socio-economic class can, on average, expect to live just over seven years longer than those in the lowest socio-economic class, and more of those years will be disability-free. Over the 20 years from 2012 to 2032, the population in England is predicted to grow by 8 million to just over 61 million, 4.5 million from natural growth (births – deaths), 3.5 million from net migration.

Reading

Demography, future trends. www.kingsfund.org.uk/projects/time-think-differently/trends-demography.

50 Correct Answer: A

Explanation: There is evidence that allowing safe wandering for people with dementia can reduce the incidence of delirium, and safe wandering in delirium may lessen the severity or duration.

Health promotion is still revenant in old age, and people may even see results sooner. Typical lifestyle advice still applies: exercise, weight control, healthy diet, no smoking and no/moderation of alcohol intake. People tend to have better healthcare outcomes if they are happy and not lonely. Social prescribing can also help older people and can help tackle social isolation and loneliness. Physical activity delays or prevents the worsening of frailty and in some situations may even reverse frailty to some extent. Generally speaking the more the better, including the use of weights when possible to build strength. Exercise may help prevent dementia, but current data to support this are limited to observational studies.

Reading

British Geriatrics Society. Healthier for longer: How healthcare professionals can support older people. 2019. www.bgs.org.uk/resources/healthier-for-longer-how-healthcare-professionals-can-support-older-people.

51 Correct Answer: E

Explanation: Smoking should be stopped at any age because this can impact on the development of frailty, falls risk and bone health. Unfortunately, the increased dementia risk is probably not reversed by stopping smoking.

Stopping smoking four weeks prior to surgery can improve outcomes. Alcohol has many potential harms, including accidents (e.g. falls), depression, poor sleep, incontinence, confusion, malnutrition, hypothermia, cancer risk, liver disease and high blood pressure. Older drinkers are less likely to binge drink than younger people are. High alcohol intake is a risk factor for developing dementia. There is uncertainty of the impact at lower intake levels, but there are no reliable data suggesting a beneficial effect.

Reading

British Geriatrics Society. Healthier for longer: How healthcare professionals can support older people. 2019. www.bgs.org.uk/resources/healthier-for-longer-how-healthcare-professionals-can-support-older-people.

52 Correct Answer: D

Explanation: Poor dental health is associated with an increased risk of aspiration pneumonia.

It has been estimated that around 20% of people in care homes are dehydrated. This is in part due to a loss of thirst sensation in old age and especially in those with dementia. For some people, fluid intake may also decline due to concerns about accessing the toilet (e.g. mobility or stairs) or concerns about precipitating an incontinence episode. There may be difficulty with teeth brushing due to motor problems (e.g. Parkinson's disease) or cognition (e.g. jaw clenching in advanced dementia). Dentures should not be worn overnight, as there is a risk that loose-fitting dentures can be swallowed.

Reading

British Geriatrics Society. Healthier for longer: How healthcare professionals can support older people. 2019. www.bgs.org.uk/resources/healthier-for-longer-how-healthcare-professionals-can-support-older-people.

53 Correct Answer: B

Explanation: This description provided in the stem refers to a chronic 'sterile' inflammation model of ageing, where chronic inflammation is known as sterile inflammation due to the lack of detectable mediators or the characteristic redness, pain, heat or swelling seen in local, acute inflammation (sometimes called 'inflammageing'). The source of this chronic inflammation has not been well defined, although candidate sources have been suggested, including diminished regulation of the immune system, oxidative stress, chronic antigenic stress and senescent cell accumulation.

Reading

Allyson K. Palmer, James L. Kirkland. Chapter 2, The biology of aging. In *Reichel's care of the elderly* (Seventh edition). Eds. Busby-Whitehead J, Arenson C, Durso SC, Swagerty D, Mosqueda L, Singh MF, Reichel W. Cambridge: Cambridge University Press, 2016. https://www.cambridge.org/core/books/reichels-care-of-the-elderly/biology-of-aging/08F4D01402A56818BAFEC20F9CD93B08

3

Chronic Disease and Disability
(Diagnosis and Management)

> **LEARNING OBJECTIVE:**
>
> To be able to diagnose and manage chronic disease and disability in older patients in both hospital and community settings, including the key geriatric syndromes and common causes of disability, and to understand the effects of appropriate interventions, including traditional medicine and social prescribing.

These can include:

- Anaemia/haematology
- Cardiovascular medicine (ischaemic heart disease, heart failure, atrial fibrillation, valve disease, hypertension)
- Dermatology
- Endocrine and metabolic medicine
- Gastroenterology
- Infection and sepsis
- Musculoskeletal medicine (including osteoarthritis, polymyalgia rheumatica, osteomalacia, Paget's disease, bone effects of thyroid disease)
- Neurology (peripheral neuropathy)
- Movement disorders (Parkinson's disease, Parkinsonism, Lewy body dementia, essential tremor, multisystem atrophy, progressive supranuclear palsy) and their significance in the context of population demography changes and other age-related diseases (including symptoms, signs, progress, complications, investigations, imaging and management of movement disorders)
- Renal medicine, including fluid/electrolyte imbalance; urology and prostate disease
- Respiratory medicine
- Sensory impairment

Other questions might concern:

- Drug and non-drug management of chronic conditions, including use of aids and appliances and technology.
- Services available to support patients and carers.

Questions

Question 54

An 82-year-old patient has recently been diagnosed with a localised solid-organ cancer. Unfortunately, due to a number of comorbidities, including heart failure and chronic lung disease, surgical resection of the tumour is not thought to be possible. The use of radiotherapy is being considered. Which of the following statements regarding radiotherapy is most likely to be correct?

A. brachytherapy has the advantage over stereotactic radiotherapy of not requiring the use of general anaesthesia

B. colonic cancer usually responds well to radiotherapy

C. hypofractionation allows higher daily doses of radiation to be delivered over fewer sessions

D. physical and cognitive impairments do not impact on the utility of radiotherapy

E. radiotherapy alone cannot cure cancer

Question 55

You review a 76-year-old woman in the outpatient clinic with poorly controlled heart failure despite good adherence to several medications prescribed for this indication. You are considering alternative therapeutic options. Ivabradine can be considered as a treatment for chronic stable heart failure in which of the following situations?

A. co-existent atrial fibrillation

B. ejection fraction 45% or less

C. heart failure with preserved ejection fraction

D. heart rate below 60 beats per minute

E. when a beta blocker is contraindicated

Question 56

An 84-year-old woman complains of a tremor affecting her right hand, which has gradually increased over the past few years. She has a number of other comorbidities that complicate her assessment, and after clinical evaluation you are unsure of the diagnosis. Which of the following investigations is most likely to assist in the diagnosis of Parkinson's disease?

A. apomorphine challenge test

B. ^{123}I-FP-CIT single photon emission computed tomography (SPECT)

C. objective smell testing

D. positron emission tomography (PET)

E. structural MRI scanning

Question 57

An 86-year-old man expresses concern that his home blood pressure recordings have been high and seeks your advice as to whether he should start blood pressure lowering medication. He lives with his wife and is independent for all of his personal care. He has no significant past medical history and currently takes no regular medications. Which criterion is the most appropriate for prescribing this man antihypertensive medication?

A. 10-year cardiovascular risk calculated as greater than 10%

B. blood pressure greater than 140/90 mmHg

C. blood pressure greater than 150/90 mmHg

D. daytime ambulatory blood pressure greater than 135/85 mmHg

E. detection of proteinuria

Question 58

A patient on your ward is prescribed multiple medications. Her family have noted a progressive cognitive decline over the last year. According to the Anticholinergic Cognitive Burden scale, which of the following drugs is associated with the highest risk of cognitive adverse effects in older people with frailty?

A. prednisolone

B. ranitidine

C. risperidone

D. solifenacin

E. trazodone

Question 59

A new drug to prevent heart failure has been tested against placebo in a randomised trial. Over the 12-month trial duration, 46 of 1,000 people in the active treatment group developed heart failure, compared to 66 of 1,000 people receiving placebo. What is the number needed to treat for one year with the new drug to prevent one case of heart failure?

A. 2

B. 20

C. 46

D. 50

E. 112

Question 60

Which of the following statements regarding medication use by older people is most likely to be correct?

A. adverse drug reactions are estimated to have a prevalence around 50% in older people at the time of an acute hospital admission

B. approximately 30% of older people continue taking bisphosphonate medications after 12 months

C. around 25% of care home residents are prescribed one or more medications classified as potentially inappropriate

D. around 50% of people in the UK aged over 80 regularly take ten or more medications

E. prescription cascades are an example of inappropriate polypharmacy

Question 61

An older person reports difficulty taking all of her multiple medications as prescribed. Her daughter asks if a multi-compartment system would be useful. Which of the following medications would be most suitable to put in a multi-compartment drug administration aid?

A. alendronate

B. co-careldopa

C. donepezil

D. tiotropium

E. warfarin

Question 62

A 71-year-old man has newly been diagnosed with Parkinson's disease in the outpatient clinic. He presented with a right-hand tremor, stiffness and slowness that had gradually increased over the past 12 months. His symptoms are now affecting his quality of life, and he is keen to start treatment but also concerned about the possible side effects of medication. You discuss with him the relative benefits and risks of treatment. Which side effect is more likely to occur with levodopa prescription rather than a dopamine agonist?

A. ankle oedema

B. daytime sleepiness

C. hallucinations

D. impulse control disorders

E. motor fluctuations

Question 63

You have been asked to help rewrite your hospital's older persons' heart failure clinic lifestyle advice sheet. Which of the following advice would best apply to all people with a diagnosis of heart failure?

A. advise not to drive

B. avoid air travel

C. offer pneumococcal vaccine

D. reduce dietary salt intake

E. reduce fluid intake

Question 64

You are reviewing a man with Parkinson's disease in the outpatient clinic. You are discussing starting him on a dopamine agonist to improve his symptom control. He has heard reports in the media of people developing problems, including compulsive gambling, on this type of treatment. He asks you to tell him more about this potential adverse effect. Which of the following statements regarding impulse control disorders is most likely to be accurate?

A. all dopaminergic medication must be withheld initially

B. cognitive behaviour therapy is the most effective treatment

C. increased risk in current smokers

D. only occurs with dopamine agonist medications

E. suggests the onset of Parkinson's disease dementia

Question 65

An 81-year-old man is reviewed in the outpatient clinic. He has been admitted three times in the last year for exacerbations of COPD and has had another two recent episodes of pneumonia. His comorbidities include ischaemic heart disease, hypertension and a non-disabling stroke. He currently uses a long-acting muscarinic dry powder inhaler and a short-acting beta-agonist as required to manage his COPD. He still smokes around ten cigarettes per day and does not want to stop. He has no childhood history of asthma. He scores well on cognitive testing and reports good adherence to his medications. Osteoarthritis changes are noted in his hands. No kyphosis, clubbing or cyanosis are present. He has mild lung hyper-expansion both on examination and on his chest X-ray. Blood tests showed his eosinophil count to be in the normal range. What change to his therapy would be most appropriate to reduce the risk of further COPD exacerbations?

A. add a long-acting beta-2 agonist dry powder inhaler

B. add an inhaled corticosteroid dry powder inhaler

C. start antibiotic prophylaxis with azithromycin

D. switch to a long-acting beta-2 agonist dry powder inhaler

E. switch to a long-acting muscarinic agonist metered dose inhaler via a spacer

Question 66

An 83-year-old woman has attended the falls clinic due to having three falls in her own home during the last three months. Her past medical history includes type 2 diabetes, chronic renal impairment and vascular dementia. She has previously had problems managing her medications. She lives alone. For diabetic control, she receives a once daily subcutaneous insulin injection that is administered by a district nurse. What would be a suitable target range for her HbA$_{1c}$?

A. 48 to 53 mmol/mol (6.5% to 7.0%)

B. 53 to 59 mmol/mol (7.0% to 7.5%)

C. 59 to 64 mmol/mol (7.5% to 8.0%)

D. 64 to 75 mmol/mol (8.0% to 9.0%)

E. 75 to 86 mmol/mol (9.0% to 10.0%)

Question 67

A 72-year-old woman has attended the outpatient clinic complaining of low mood and constipation. Her only significant past history is a diagnosis of rheumatoid arthritis, for which she is taking oral methotrexate. As part of her assessment, some blood tests were taken to assess her thyroid function, the results of which are shown below:

TABLE 3.1

Investigations.

Serum thyroid-Stimulating hormone	9.5 mIU/L (0.30–4.50)
Free T4	12.1 pmol/L (10.0–22.0)

What would be the most appropriate response to these blood test results?

A. measure serum free T3 concentration

B. repeat thyroid blood tests in six weeks

C. start levothyroxine 25 mcg once daily

D. start levothyroxine 50 mcg once daily

E. test for thyroid peroxidase antibodies

Question 68

The relative of a patient with Parkinson's disease asks you how common the condition is. Which of the following options is the most accurate estimate of the prevalence of Parkinson's disease in the UK population?

A. 10 people per 100,000

B. 80 people per 100,000

C. 110 people per 100,000

D. 160 people per 100,000

E. 270 people per 100,000

Question 69

A 75-year-old woman is being assessed in the falls clinic. She reports a gradual reduction in her vision over the last year. She has noticed difficulty recognising familiar faces and now struggles with reading books. She does not have any pain and has not noticed any redness of her eyes. She lives alone and is independent. She does not drink alcohol but smokes around 15 cigarettes per day. Her past medical history includes osteoarthritis and hypertension. Her only medication is amlodipine 5 mg daily. Which investigation is most likely to be helpful with diagnosis of her visual problem?

A. intraocular pressure testing

B. MRI brain scan

C. serum HbA$_{1C}$

D. slit-lamp fundus examination

E. Snellen chart test

Question 70

The local community nursing team are looking for ways to reduce antibiotic use in your region. They ask you, which intervention would be most likely to help reduce recurrent UTI diagnosis in care home residents?

A. cranberry juice

B. *D*-mannose

C. improved hydration

D. methenamine

E. vaginal oestrogens

Question 71

An 83-year-old man presents to the outpatient clinic with respiratory symptoms and reports a past history of bronchiectasis. Comparing older people with bronchiectasis to younger people with this condition, which of the following is most likely to be correct?

A. fewer cases have an idiopathic aetiology

B. greater proportion with chronic *P. aeruginosa* infection

C. higher probability of two or more exacerbations per year

D. less frequently report chronic cough

E. less likely to have underlying ciliary dysfunction

Question 72

A 71-year-old man presents with a two-year history of progressive cough, fatigue and shortness of breath on exertion. He was previously employed as an accountant but retired several years ago. He lives with his wife, is independent in self-care, has never smoked and keeps no pets. He has no relevant past medical history and takes no medications. Physical examination reveals bi-basal lung crackles only. A high-resolution CT scan of the chest showed bi-basal honeycomb changes with reticulation and traction bronchiectasis. Which treatment would be most suitable?

A. anticoagulation

B. azathioprine

C. N-acetylcysteine

D. pirfenidone

E. prednisolone

Question 73

A 67-year-old man who is living with HIV infection is admitted to your ward. Regarding older people living with HIV and prescribed antiretroviral therapy, which the following statements is most likely to be correct?

A. bisphosphonates are ineffective for treating osteoporosis related to antiretroviral drug adverse effects

B. falls risk is increased compared to people of a similar age without HIV

C. less than 5% of new infections in the developed world occur after the age of 50

D. neurocognitive impairment typically affects language ability

E. the prevalence of frailty is similar to people of a similar age without HIV

Question 74

A 70-year-old man with Parkinson's disease is reviewed in the clinic along with his wife. Although his own symptoms are currently well controlled, his wife complains that he has been lashing out at her with his arms and legs while they are asleep in bed at night. This has caused her a great deal of distress and bruising. She has now started sleeping in the spare bedroom. Which treatment would you consider prescribing?

A. melatonin

B. midodrine

C. modafinil

D. quetiapine

E. rotigotine patch

Question 75

A 74-year-old woman presents with malaise that developed over the last few weeks. Blood tests sent by her GP revealed an elevated ESR at 84 mm/hour (normal <42). A diagnosis of giant cell arteritis is suspected. Which of the following features would be more suggestive of large vessel, rather than cranial vessel, involvement?

A. abnormal temporal artery ultrasound

B. amaurosis fugax

C. diplopia

D. jaw claudication

E. pyrexia of unknown origin

Question 76

An 80-year-old man has been on apixaban for the treatment of a proximal left leg deep vein thrombosis that occurred following a fall and a fractured left hip several weeks ago. He has now returned to being independently mobile. His past medical history is of hypertension and ischaemic heart disease. Along with apixaban, he is currently taking atorvastatin 40 mg od, lisinopril 5 mg od and bisoprolol 5 mg od. Physical examination is unremarkable. His blood pressure is 128/76 mmHg, and an ECG shows sinus rhythm with a rate of 68 beats per minute. What duration of anticoagulation would be most appropriate?

A. 3 months

B. 6 months

C. 12 months

D. 24 months

E. lifelong

Question 77

You review a 75-year-old woman with Parkinson's disease in the outpatient clinic. Overall, her symptoms are reasonably well controlled and she continues to live alone independently. However, she complains of continual drooling of saliva. She finds this very embarrassing and it is causing her to limit her social engagements. Which treatment for drooling should be offered first?

A. amitriptyline

B. botulinum toxin A injections

C. glycopyrronium bromide

D. speech and language therapy

E. topical atropine

Question 78

The NHS has an abdominal aortic aneurysm (AAA) screening program that targets men aged over 66 and women aged over 70 with relevant risk factors to undergo aortic ultrasound evaluation. Which of the following comorbidities would make referral appropriate?

A. atrial fibrillation

B. chronic kidney disease

C. chronic obstructive pulmonary disease

D. fatty liver disease (NAFLD)

E. type 2 diabetes

Question 79

An 87-year-old woman was diagnosed with Parkinson's disease seven years ago. She had initially responded well to levodopa therapy but over the last year is having increasing problems with motor fluctuations that are affecting her quality of life. Which medication is the most appropriate to add to levodopa when the main aim is to achieve the greatest reduction in off time?

A. amantadine

B. cabergoline

C. entacapone

D. rasagiline

E. ropinirole

Question 80

A 74-year-old woman is referred to the outpatient clinic with pain in her arms and functional decline. She describes progression of the pain over the last three weeks with no prior history of similar symptoms. She describes stiffness lasting over an hour each morning. On examination there is evidence of inflammation around both wrist and several metacarpophalangeal joints. Blood tests from her GP showed a mild normocytic anaemia and an elevated C-reactive protein concentration. Which investigation would be most appropriate to do first?

A. aspiration of synovial fluid from a wrist

B. serum anti-cyclic citrullinated peptide antibodies

C. serum rheumatoid factor

D. ultrasound scan of the wrists

E. X-rays of both wrists

Question 81

A 70-year-old man is referred to the outpatient clinic for help with the management of severe back pain. He has had pain in his back for more than five years and has previously been seen in a spinal clinic. The source of the pain is felt to be osteoarthritis of the spine and no surgical intervention was felt to be useful. He is currently taking regular paracetamol and morphine sulphate 40 mg bd. Which of the following statements about the management of this pain is most accurate?

A. duloxetine has evidence of efficacy for chronic back pain

B. lidocaine patch should be tried

C. morphine is more effective than non-opioid drugs for chronic musculoskeletal pain control

D. pregabalin is a useful option

E. there is no evidence to suggest topical NSAIDs are superior to placebo

Question 82

Regarding people aged 80 years with a diagnosis of heart failure in the developed world, which statement is most likely to be correct?

A. around 40% of new diagnoses have a preserved ejection fraction

B. diastolic heart failure has a worse prognosis than systolic heart failure

C. one-year mortality rates are around 20%

D. the age-adjusted incidence has risen over the past ten years

E. there is an associated reduction in the duration of cardiac contraction

Question 83

An 80-year-old woman admitted to your unit is found to have advanced chronic kidney disease. Her comorbidities include COPD, hypertension, ischaemic heart disease and type 2 diabetes. Compared to a conservative management strategy, what benefit might be expected

from commencing renal replacement therapy for an older person with multiple comorbidities?

A. better symptom control

B. greater probability of dying in their own home

C. improved five-year survival rate

D. improved quality of life

E. spending less time in hospital

Question 84

Which of the following statements is most likely to be true regarding chronic kidney disease in older people with mild to moderate frailty?

A. an estimated glomerular filtration rate below 60 mL/min/1.73 m^2 usually indicates underlying renal disease

B. arterio-venous fistula formation has a lower success rate

C. atherosclerosis is the main pathological process resulting in declining renal function

D. in people with cognitive impairment, peritoneal dialysis is better tolerated than haemodialysis

E. peritoneal dialysis is more commonly used than haemodialysis

Question 85

A 72-year-old man, originally from Italy, has been found to have abnormal liver blood tests following an annual health check at his GP surgery. He does not report any symptoms. On subsequent testing, he was positive for hepatitis C virus RNA in his blood and a liver ultrasound scan suggested hepatic cirrhosis. Which of the following statements is correct?

A. annual screening for hepatocellular carcinoma with liver ultrasound is recommended

B. anti-viral treatment has not been shown to be effective in people aged over 65

C. asymptomatic infection is uncommon

D. he has around a 4% chance of developing hepatocellular carcinoma over the next year

E. he has around a 75% chance of developing end-stage liver disease

Question 86

A 69-year-old woman is seen in the outpatient clinic complaining of fatigue over the last few months. She has a past history of rheumatoid arthritis and hypertension. She currently takes clopidogrel 75 mg od, lansoprazole 30 mg od, diclofenac 50 mg tds and amlodipine 5 mg od. She does not smoke or drink alcohol. On examination, she has mild jaundice but no palpable liver, ascites or peripheral oedema.

Blood tests are as below:

TABLE 3.2

Investigations.

Bilirubin	32 μmol/L (<21)
Serum alkaline phosphatase	185 U/L (30–130)
Serum alanine transaminase	164 U/L (<40)
Globulins	41 g/L (20–35)
Hepatitis screen	Negative
Antinuclear antibody	Positive, 1:80
Anti-smooth muscle antibody	Positive, 1:40
Ultrasound of abdomen	No hepatobiliary abnormality

Which action would be most appropriate to do next?

A. change diclofenac to an alternative analgesic

B. echocardiogram

C. liver biopsy

D. serum paraprotein and urinary light chain evaluation

E. start oral prednisolone 60 mg daily

Question 87

You review a 70-year-old woman with a long history of constipation. She has no other significant past medical history and her only current medication is a combination of stimulant and osmotic laxatives. She has been seen in a constipation specialist clinic and underwent a number of tests. Following this, she is commenced on a programme of biofeedback training. What is the most likely cause of this woman's constipation?

A. amyloidosis

B. dyssynergistic defaecation

C. Hirchsprung disease

D. irritable bowel syndrome

E. slow-transit constipation

Question 88

A 79-year-old man presents with a rash. He reports a two-month history of generalised itching but over the last two weeks he has also noticed blistering of his skin. He has a past history of COPD, ischaemic heart disease, type 2 diabetes and a lacunar stroke two years ago. He regularly takes aspirin, metformin, atorvastatin, bisoprolol and a tiotropium inhaler. On examination, he has tense blisters, approximately 2 cm in diameter affecting the flexor aspects of his arms and legs and across his lower abdomen. What is the most likely diagnosis?

A. bullous pemphigoid

B. cutaneous drug reaction

C. dermatitis herpetiformis

D. pemphigus vulgaris

E. systemic varicella zoster

Question 89

A 77-year-old woman of South Asian heritage is reviewed in the outpatient clinic. She has had persistently elevated blood pressure readings both in primary care and at a prior clinic visit. An ambulatory blood pressure reading showed an average daytime blood pressure of 162/93 mmHg. She usually lives alone independently. She has no significant past medical history and currently takes no regular medications. Physical examination reveals a soft pan systolic heart murmur, clear lungs and bilateral pitting ankle oedema. She is keen to start medication to reduce her future risk of vascular disease. Which initial drug type would you advise to treat her hypertension?

A. angiotensin converting enzyme inhibitor
B. angiotensin receptor blocker
C. beta blocker
D. calcium channel blocker
E. thiazide-like diuretic

Question 90

An 87-year-old man complains of increased urinary frequency with urgency and nocturia four times each night. He also describes a poor urinary flow with hesitancy before starting to pass urine. These symptoms have slowly developed over the last year or two. His past medical history includes severe depression, for which he takes a combination of sertraline and mirtazapine. Physical examination reveals an enlarged but smooth prostate. He is found to have a postural drop in his blood pressure falling from 146/83 mmHg when lying to 135/79 mmHg on standing. A post-void bladder scan reveals a residual urine volume of 296 mls. He is very keen to avoid urinary catheterisation or any surgical procedure.

Which treatment would you recommend for him?

A. doxazosin
B. finasteride
C. mirabegron
D. solifenacin
E. tamsulosin

Question 91

A 72-year-old man has recently been diagnosed with heart failure. An echocardiogram estimated his ejection fraction to be 34%. He also has type 2 diabetes. Which medication may be beneficial for the control of both his heart failure and diabetes?

A. dapagliflozin
B. gliclazide
C. liraglutide
D. pioglitazone
E. sitagliptin

Question 92

A 73-year-old man complains of increasing pain in his legs and pelvis over the last few months. Initial blood tests showed a raised serum alkaline phosphatase concentration. Which X-ray abnormality would be most consistent with a diagnosis of Paget's disease?

A. avascular necrosis
B. chondrocalcinosis
C. joint space narrowing
D. loss of distinction between the cortex and medulla
E. trabecular thinning

Question 93

An 86-year-old woman was admitted to hospital after presenting to the emergency department with shortness of breath, productive cough and palpitations. A chest X-ray demonstrated a left lower lobe pneumonia, and an electrocardiogram showed atrial fibrillation with a fast ventricular response.

To investigate for an underlying cause of atrial fibrillation, thyroid function tests were added to blood tests from admission, with results as listed below.

What is the most appropriate next investigation to further evaluate these thyroid function tests?

TABLE 3.3

Investigations.

Serum thyroid-stimulating hormone	0.4 mU/L (0.4–5)
Free serum T$_4$	14.1 pmol/L (10–22)
Free serum T$_3$	4.4 pmol/L (5–10)

A. repeat thyroid function tests in six weeks

B. thyroglobulin antibody levels

C. thyroid peroxidase antibody levels

D. thyroid scintiscanning

E. thyroid ultrasound

Question 94

A 66-year-old man is seeing his GP after a routine health review. He is independent and lives most of the year in Mexico. The only symptom he reports is of fatigue. He is obese and has hypertension and type 2 diabetes for which he takes amlodipine and metformin. He smokes around six cigarettes a day, drinks around 20 units of alcohol a week and is a retired architect. On examination, he has a soft abdomen with no masses. His chest is clear, and there is no scleral icterus or pallor. He is well tanned and his body mass index is 30 kg/m².

The GP completes routine bloods as below.

What is the cause of the metabolic derangement?

Table 3.4

Investigations.

Serum sodium	140 mmol/L (137–144)
Serum potassium	4.5 mmol/L (3.5–4.9)
Serum urea	5.6 mmol/L (2.5–7.5)
Serum creatinine	92 μmol/L (60–110)
Haemoglobin	145 g/dL (130–180 g/L)
Platelet count	355 × 10⁹/L (150–400)
White cell count	9.4 × 10⁹/L (4–11)
Serum total bilirubin	17 μmol/L (1–22)
Serum alanine aminotransferase	107 u/L (5–35)
Serum aspartate aminotransferase	80 u/L (1–31)
Serum alkaline phosphatase	122 u/L (45–105)
Serum gamma glutamyl transferase	80 u/L (<50 U/L)
Serum albumin	36 g/L (37–49)
Ultrasound liver	Increased hepatic echogenicity

A. alcoholic fatty liver disease

B. gallstones

C. haemochromatosis

D. non-alcoholic fatty liver disease

E. Wilson's disease

Question 95

An 82-year-old man with metastatic lung carcinoma presents with increasing lethargy and a number of falls. He describes feeling light-headed on standing from his bed. His appetite has been poor, he feels lethargic and he has vomited twice daily for the past three days. Medications include omeprazole for mild reflux symptoms. On examination, he has a tanned complexion and cachexia. Capillary refill time is prolonged to four seconds. He appears pale with dry mucosa and his abdomen is soft and non-tender. There are reduced breath sounds at both lung bases, which are both dull to percussion.

TABLE 3.5

Investigations.

Serum sodium	127 mmol/L (137–144)
Serum potassium	5.1 mmol/L (3.5–4.9)
Serum urea	7.5 mmol/L (2.5–7.5)
Serum creatinine	94 μmol/L (60–110)
Serum CRP	35 mg/L (<10)
Haemoglobin	99 g/L (130–180)
White cell count	6.0×10^9/L (4.0–11.0)
Neutrophil count	5.2×10^9/L (1.5–7.0)
Lymphocyte count	0.8×10^9/L (1.5–4)
Cosinophil count	0.2×10^9/L (0.04–0.4)
Platelet count	240×10^9/L (150–400)
CT chest, abdomen and pelvis	There is a 4-1/2 cm mass in the right lower lobe, with extension to adjacent pleura. Bilateral pleural effusions are present. There is mediastinal lymphadenopathy and enlargement of para-aortic nodes with masses seen in both adrenals. Findings are in keeping with a primary lung malignancy with metastatic spread.

Blood pressure is 95/69 mmHg, heart rate 88/min, respiratory rate 26/min.

What is the likeliest explanation of this presentation?

A. Addisonian crisis

B. pneumonia

C. progressive dwindling

D. proton pump inhibitor adverse effects

E. syndrome of inappropriate anti-diuretic hormone (SIADH)

Question 96

A 76-year-old retired farmer presents with a four-week history of increasing shortness of breath, non-specific non-pleuritic chest pain and weight loss. He is known to keep racing pigeons in a small shed. He keeps active, lives alone, drinks a moderate amount of alcohol and is a life-long smoker with a 40 pack/year history. He has no known allergies. On examination, you note bilateral finger clubbing and tar staining. Respiratory examination revealed a respiratory rate of 19 breaths per minute, oxygen saturation 94% on air, reduced bilateral chest expansion and reduced air entry in both bases associated with dullness to percussion.

Investigations

What is the most appropriate next investigation?

A. bronchoscopy with bronchoalveolar lavage

B. chest drain

C. CT chest/abdomen/pelvis with contrast

D. high-resolution CT chest

E. video-assisted thoracoscopic biopsy

TABLE 3.6

Investigations.

Chest X-ray	Moderate right > left bilateral pleural effusions and patchy opacities across both lung fields in a non-lobar distribution
High-resolution lung CT	Small bilateral pleural effusion, thickened pleura with no lung parenchymal abnormalities
Lung function testing	FEV_1 1.9L, FVC 52% of predicted value

TABLE 3.7

Investigations.

Arterial blood gases on air:	
PaO$_2$	7.2 kPa (11.3–12.6)
PCO$_2$	5.2 kPa (4.7–6.0)
pH	7.38 (7.35–7.45)
HCO$_3$	26 mmol/L (21–29)

Arterial blood gases after one litre of O$_2$ per minute via a nasal cannula:	
PaO$_2$	9.5 kPa (11.3–12.6)
PCO$_2$	6.8 kPa (4.7–6.0)
pH	7.23 (7.35–7.45)
HCO$_3$	28 mmol/L (21–29)

Question 97

You arrange a long-term oxygen therapy (LTOT) assessment for a 69-year-old man. He has a past medical history of severe chronic obstructive pulmonary disease. He has developed dyspnoea at rest. He has no risk factors for falls or sustaining burns.

Results of the LTOT assessment are as follows:

The patient feels less short of breath at the end of the trial. How will you manage this patient?

A. bi-level positive airway pressure ('BiPAP')

B. continuous positive airway pressure ('CPAP')

C. decline LTOT

D. further medical optimisation and reassess after four weeks

E. provide LTOT

Question 98

A 67-year-old male presents to the neurology clinic with his wife, reporting a three-month history of worsening vision in his left eye. Over the past two months, he has had a constant and increasing headache, worse at night and on coughing. He has occasionally felt extremely nauseated and vomited several times, at least twice waking him from sleep. His wife also notes significant personality change. She notes that he has become increasingly emotional. Prior to these symptoms, he has been fit and well with no past medical or drug history. On examination, you note a left relative afferent papillary defect with equally sized pupils. Specialist examination is then performed in a local eye clinic. Visual acuity in the left eye is 6/60 and 6/9 on the right. Testing of colour vision with Ishihara plates demonstrates 0/17 on the left and 17/17 on the right. A central scotoma is found in the left eye. Fundoscopy of the left eye reveals a pale optic disc with poor vasculature while the right appears swollen. A full range of painless eye movements is demonstrated, and cranial nerve examination is normal. What is the most likely diagnosis?

A. age-related macular degeneration

B. Foster-Kennedy syndrome

C. frontotemporal dementia

D. idiopathic intracranial hypertension

E. multiple sclerosis

Question 99

A 78-year-old man presents with chronic pelvic pain and voiding symptoms, in the absence of a urinary tract syndrome. The doctor explains to him that the cause is often not fully understood, but he is given a diagnosis of chronic bacterial prostatitis/chronic pelvic pain syndrome. His pain is neuropathic in nature, and a nociceptive/inflammatory aetiology is not suspected. What is the next best management step?

A. continue non-steroidal anti-inflammatory drugs

B. continue paracetamol

C. discontinue non-steroidal anti-inflammatory drugs and paracetamol, and consider capsaicin cream first line according to the clinical situation

D. discontinue non-steroidal anti-inflammatory drugs and paracetamol, and consider tramadol first line according to the clinical situation

E. discontinue non-steroidal anti-inflammatory drugs and paracetamol, offer a choice of amitriptyline, duloxetine, gabapentin or pregabalin according to the clinical situation and refer him to pain specialists following a multidisciplinary team discussion

Question 100

A 92-year-old resident of a nursing home, with advanced dementia, complains of a three-month history of a widespread hyperkeratotic dermatosis, typically involving the palms and soles, with deep skin fissures, and generalised lymphadenopathy. On reflection, according to nursing notes, this had probably developed over several months. Other known problems had been the emergence of 'shouting out' at nighttime, only in the last few months. Blood results reveal peripheral blood eosinophilia and raised serum IgE levels. A diagnosis of crusted scabies is made. The diagnosis has been delayed in part due to the communication difficulties with the resident. It is decided to adopt an approach to management which includes eradication of mites, management of symptoms and complications, and treatment of close contacts to minimise transmission. What chemical intervention would be considered first line?

A. benzoyl benzoate

B. crotamiton

C. malathion

D. permethrin, 5% cream

E. sulphur

Question 101

An older person has been prescribed antibiotics for the outpatient management of cellulitis. You should also advise about seeking medical help if symptoms worsen rapidly or significantly at any time or do not start to improve within what time frame?

A. two to three days

B. four to five days

C. six to seven days

D. after a week

E. after a month

Question 102

A 79-year-old woman is admitted with a two-month history of malaise and lethargy. She denies any weight loss, abdominal pain or bloating, altered bowel habit or bleeding per rectally. She has experienced no abnormal menopausal bleeding. She has no family history of coeliac disease. On admission she looks comfortable. Her abdominal examination is normal.

Which of the following is the most appropriate next step?

A. CT abdomen
B. endoscopy and colonoscopy
C. faecal occult blood testing
D. transferrin saturation evaluation
E. transfuse two units of blood

Answers for Chapter 3

54 Correct Answer: C

Explanation: External beam radiotherapy uses high-energy X-ray beams to cause DNA damage within cancer cells, aiming to avoid surrounding tissues as much as possible. Cancer cells are believed to have reduced DNA repair mechanisms and so become more susceptible to radiation damage. It is delivered in a number of daily doses (fractions). Hypofractionation is a term for giving higher doses of radiotherapy over a smaller number of sessions. Palliative courses usually last one day to two weeks, whereas curative treatments may last up to eight weeks. It can be used with chemotherapy concurrently or sequentially. Treatment sites are marked with permanent tattoos. Recipients must lie still, typically for five- to ten-minute periods, and sometimes hold their breath temporarily, which may limit its use in people with cognitive impairment. Recipients usually need to be able to transfer from bed to couch with assistance. Modern techniques include linear accelerators and stereotactic radiotherapy (higher dose with more localised delivery). Brachytherapy is a localised treatment involving applying the radiation source directly onto the tumour, usually under general anaesthetic. This technique is useful for some prostate, cervical, endometrial, rectal and skin cancers.

Side effects of radiotherapy include fatigue and local tissue irritation. Short-term changes (within the first three months) relate to tissue inflammation (e.g. pain) and usually improve over a few weeks. Long-term complications include fibrosis, alternations to blood supply and a small risk of secondary malignancies. Older people seem to tolerate radiotherapy similarly to younger people. Brain radiotherapy may increase the risk of cognitive impairment. The incidence of side effects can be reduced by more precise modern techniques (e.g. intensity modulated radiotherapy [IMRT] and volumetric modulated arc therapy [VMAT]). Also, improved imaging techniques guide treatment more accurately to the right location.

Currently, it is used in around 40% of curative cancer treatment regimens, and 16% of cancers can be cured by radiotherapy alone (usually in the absence of metastatic disease, examples include some lung, prostate, bladder, oesophagus, head/neck and non-melanotic skin cancers). It is particularly useful for older people in non-melanoma skin cancers. Large bowel cancers, other than rectal cancer, do not usually respond well to radiotherapy. Palliative radiotherapy can help with pain control (e.g. bone metastases), tumour shrinkage (e.g. cerebral metastases or spinal cord compression), haemorrhage, dysphagia and cough symptoms.

Reading

Cree A, O'Donovan, O'Hanlon S. New horizons in radiotherapy for older people. *Age Ageing* 2019; 48: 605–612.

TABLE 3.8

Investigations.

Haemoglobin	90 g/L (130–180)
MCV	66 fL (80–96)
Serum ferritin	8 µg/L (15–300)
Coeliac screen	Normal

55 Correct Answer: E

Explanation: Ivabradine is currently recommended for people with New York Heart Association (NYHA) class II to IV stable chronic heart failure with systolic dysfunction (ejection fraction 35% or less) and in sinus rhythm with a heart rate of 75 beats per minute or more. Ivabradine is given in combination with standard therapy including beta blocker, angiotensin-converting enzyme (ACE) inhibitor and aldosterone antagonist, or when beta-blocker therapy is contraindicated or not tolerated. It should be started by a heart failure specialist.

Reading

National Institute for Health and Care Excellence. Chronic heart failure in adults: Diagnosis and management. 2018. www.nice.org.uk/guidance/ng106.

56 Correct Answer: B

Explanation: ^{123}I-FP-CIT single photon emission computed tomography (SPECT) is sometimes used to help distinguish essential tremor from Parkinson's disease when not clear from clinical features alone. The other testing options have been evaluated but are not currently recommended in clinical practice.

Reading

National Institute for Health and Care Excellence. Parkinson's disease in adults. 2017. www.nice.org.uk/guidance/ng71.

57 Correct Answer: C

Explanation: The description is of a non-frail, non-multimorbid person aged over 80 with stage 1 hypertension. Current guidance is to offer treatment for people aged over 80 years if the clinic blood pressure is over 150/90 mmHg (both standing and seated BP measurements should be taken—use the lower value if significant drop or if postural hypotension symptoms). The daytime ambulatory/home BP monitor target should be below 145/85 mmHg. All people with stage 2 hypertension should be considered for treatment. Consider drug treatment in people aged <60 even with a ten-year cardiovascular risk <10%. Offer treatment when age <80 if stage 1 hypertension plus one of the following: target organ damage, cardiovascular disease, renal disease, diabetes or ten-year cardiovascular risk >10%. Proteinuria can be a sign of target organ damage when associated with elevated blood pressure but would not be criteria for prescribing treatment alone. Target organ damage can affect the heart, brain, kidneys and eyes. Examples are left ventricular hypertrophy, chronic kidney disease, hypertensive retinopathy and increased urine albumin to creatinine ratio. Test for proteinuria, look at fundi, do an ECG, test urea and electrolytes (U&Es).

Reading

National Institute for Health and Care Excellence. Hypertension in adults: Diagnosis and management. Guideline 136, 2019. www.nice.org.uk/guidance/ng136.

58 Correct Answer: D

Explanation: A number of anticholinergic adverse effect scales have been developed. Unfortunately, due to differing methods, there is some degree of variation between the scales. On the

Anticholinergic Cognitive Burden scale, solifenacin has a score of 3, whereas the other drugs in this question are all rated as 1.

Reading

Salahudeen MS, Duffull SB, Nishtala PS. Anticholinergic burden quantified by anticholinergic risk scales and adverse outcomes in older people: A systematic review. *BMC Geriatrics* 2015; 15: 31.

59 Correct Answer: D

Number needed to treat (NNT) = 100 divided by absolute risk reduction (ARR) as a percentage.

ARR = event rate on placebo minus event rate on active drug = (66/1000) − (46/1000) = 20/1000 = 2/100 = 2%

NNT = 100/2 = 50

60 Correct Answer: E

Explanation: Adverse drug reactions are thought to be present in around 10% of older people at the time of acute hospital admission (but the true value may be higher if the reactions present in an atypical way). The 12-month adherence rates for statins and bisphosphonates are around 60%–70%, but the value is around 35% for bladder anticholinergics (although the use of dosette boxes may affect the selective ability for some older people). Around 35%–60% of care home residents are estimated to be prescribed one or more potentially inappropriate medications (PIMs) (and around 30% of older people living in their own home). Currently in the UK, around 25% of people aged over 80 regularly take ten or more medications. Examples of inappropriate polypharmacy include hazardous or interacting drug combinations, ineffective drugs, unacceptable therapeutic burden, presence of reduced adherence and prescription cascades.

Reading

Woodford HJ, Fisher J. New horizons in deprescribing for older people. *Age Ageing* 2019; 48: 768–775.

61 Correct Answer: C

Explanation: Monitored dosage systems (also referred to as multi-compartment compliance aids, dosette boxes or blister packs) are intended to make it easier for people to adhere to treatments, especially in association with polypharmacy. However, many drugs cannot be placed within them, which can actually increase complexity. They can help to administer regular solid oral medications at a stable dose (i.e. not warfarin, insulin, liquids, suppositories, inhalers, creams, eye drops, patches or 'as required' drugs). They are also less suitable for people with complex drug timings such as in Parkinson's disease or medications that need to be taken in a specific way (e.g. bisphosphonates). Taking medicines out of their original packaging can introduce moisture and is not suitable for soluble or buccal absorption formulations. They might be more useful for people with cognitive, vision or dexterity impairment.

Reading

Duerden M. What is the place for monitored dosage systems? *Drug Therap Bull* 2018; 56: 102–106.

62 Correct Answer: E

Explanation: Levodopa use results in better motor improvement and quality of life compared to dopamine agonists but with a risk of longer-term motor complications, including dyskinesia and fluctuations. Side effects of dopamine agonists include hallucinations, ankle oedema, daytime sleepiness and impulse control disorders.

Reading

National Institute for Health and Care Excellence. Parkinson's disease in adults. 2017. www.nice.org. uk/guidance/ng71.

63 Correct Answer: C

Reducing fluid intake is only advised if there is dilutional hyponatraemia. Reduce dietary salt only if intake is excessive (also avoid replacing with potassium-containing salt substitutes). Air travel is usually possible. It should not affect driving ability in the early stages (see Driver and Vehicle Licensing Agency [DVLA] for UK advice). Pneumococcal vaccination (once) and annual influenza immunisation are recommended.

Reading

National Institute for Health and Care Excellence. Chronic heart failure in adults: Diagnosis and management. 2018. www.nice.org.uk/guidance/ng106.

64 Correct Answer: C

Explanation: Recognised risk factors for developing impulse control disorders include current alcohol use, current smoker, dopamine agonist prescription and prior impulsive behaviour pattern. The risk is greatest with dopamine agonists but can occur with other dopaminergic therapies. Different types of behaviour have been reported, including compulsive gambling, hypersexuality, binge eating and obsessive shopping. The person may try to conceal this behaviour. Patients and family/carers should be warned of the potential risk when starting treatment. Its occurrence is likely to result in dopaminergic drug dose reduction and possible discontinuation of any dopamine agonist drug. Cognitive behavioural therapy may also be tried if drug adjustments alone do not resolve the problem.

Reading

National Institute for Health and Care Excellence. Parkinson's disease in adults. 2017. www.nice.org. uk/guidance/ng71.

65 Correct Answer: A

Explanation: Long-acting beta-2 agonists have been shown to reduce exacerbations of COPD and are suitable to use in combination with long-acting muscarinic drugs (a single inhaler containing both drugs may be even better). The risk of cardiac toxicity appears to be very low. The dry powder formulation seems a sensible one for the described man. Switching to a metered dose inhaler via a spacer may help if force of inspiration were markedly reduced. The presence of only mild chest hyper-expansion is against this. Patients tend to find spacers more of a burden to use and it would require re-education in the different inhaler technique. Corticosteroids would increase the risk of this man developing further pneumonia, and there are no indicators that he would benefit (i.e. no history of asthma and normal eosinophil count). Azithromycin is not recommended for people who currently smoke.

Reading

Global Initiative for Chronic Obstructive Lung Disease. Global strategy for the diagnosis, management, and prevention of chronic obstructive pulmonary disease. 2020. www.goldcopd.org.

66 Correct Answer: D

Explanation: The typical target range for younger adults with type 2 diabetes is 53 to 59 mmol/mol. Sometimes a lower target is set for people on diet control alone or minimal oral drug therapy. However, in older people with frailty, the risk of hypoglycaemia increases. The scenario describes a very vulnerable woman.

Individualised and more lenient targets are appropriate for those at greatest risk of hypoglycaemia. A target of 59 to 64 mmol/mol (7.5% to 8.0%) may be suitable for non-frail older people and a target of 64 to 75 mmol/mol (8.0% to 9.0%) for those with frailty. Metabolic decompensation with cachexia is unlikely below the 75 mmol/mol (9.0%) level.

Reading

National Institute for Health and Care Excellence. Type 2 diabetes in adults: Management. 2015. www. nice.org.uk/guidance/ng28.

Sherman FT. Tight blood glucose control and cardiovascular disease in the elderly diabetic? *Geriatrics* 2008; 63 (8): 8–10.

67 Correct Answer: E

Explanation: This woman has subclinical hypothyroidism (TSH high, fT4 in normal range). Treatment with levothyroxine is not recommended in this scenario, i.e. TSH less than 10 with fT4 in the normal range. A measurement of fT3 is useful when TSH is low. Repeating the blood tests in six weeks would be ok; however, given this woman's history of autoimmune disease, testing for thyroid peroxidase antibodies is typically recommended.

Reading

National Institute for Health and Care Excellence. Thyroid disease: Assessment and management. 2019. www.nice.org.uk/guidance/ng145.

68 Correct Answer: D

Explanation: Parkinson's disease is one of the commonest neurological conditions. Prevalence in the UK is estimated to be around 160 people per 100,000, and the incidence is around 15–20 per 100,000 per year.

Reading

National Institute for Health and Care Excellence. Parkinson's disease in adults. 2017. www.nice.org.uk/guidance/ng71.

69 Correct Answer: D

Explanation: Age-related macular degeneration (ARMD) is the commonest cause of visual loss in the developed world. Prevalence in the UK is estimated to be 4.8% of people aged over 65 and 12.2% of people aged over 80. It causes painless visual impairment mainly affecting the central aspect of vision, often noticed as difficulty recognising faces or when reading. Diagnosis is aided by slit-lamp biomicroscopic fundus examination. Larger Drusen and more retinal pigmentation are associated with greater risk of progression to visual loss. Late forms of AMD include the 'wet' type associated with neovascularisation and the 'dry' form associated with atrophy. Risk factors include older age, family history of AMD, smoking, hypertension, BMI 30 kg/m^2 or over, diet high in fat and low level of exercise. Optical coherence tomography (OCT) is performed for people with suspected late wet AMD. This group of people should be referred to an ophthalmologist for consideration of anti-angiogenic therapies, i.e. intravitreal anti-vascular endothelial growth factor (VEGF) treatment.

Reading

National Institute for Health and Care Excellence. Age-related macular degeneration. 2018. www.nice.org.uk/guidance/ng82.

70 Correct Answer: C

Explanation: Improving hydration of care home residents seems to reduce the incidence of UTI diagnosis (possibly through reducing misdiagnosis of dark/ smelly urine and functional decline due to dehydration). Cranberry juice, *D*-mannose and methenamine have not been shown to be effective in care home residents. There is limited evidence for a rôle on vaginal oestrogens (but not oral) in reducing UTI diagnosis in non-frail women, but they are associated with significant adverse effects, are not recommended for long-term use and have low patient acceptance.

Reading

Chwa A, Kavanagh K, Linnebur SA, et al. Evaluation of methenamine for urinary tract infection prevention in older adults: A review of the evidence. *Ther Adv Drug Saf* 2019; 10: 1–9.

Lean K, Nawaz RF, Jawad S, et al. Reducing urinary tract infections in care homes by improving hydration. *BMJ Open Qual* 2019; 8: e000563.

Perrotta C, Aznar M, Mejia R, et al. Oestrogens for preventing recurrent urinary tract infection in postmenopausal women. *Cochrane Database Syst Rev* 2008; (2). Art. No.: CD005131.

71 Correct Answer: E

Explanation: The prevalence of chronic cough, sputum production and prior haemoptysis are similar among younger and older groups with bronchiectasis. An idiopathic aetiology is the most common at all ages (around 35%). Older people are more likely to have associated COPD but less likely to have ciliary dysfunction than younger people are. The prevalence of chronic infection with *P. aeruginosa* is similar at all ages (around 15%). Around 40% of people in all age groups have two or more exacerbations per year. Older people with bronchiectasis are more likely to have other comorbidities and have higher mortality rates.

Reading

Bellelli G, Chalmers JD, Sotgiu G, et al. Characterization of bronchiectasis in the elderly. *Resp Med* 2016; 119: 13–19.

72 Correct Answer: D

Explanation: The scenario describes a presentation with idiopathic pulmonary fibrosis. Pirfenidone is an anti-fibrotic drug that appears to slow lung function decline in people with this condition. The other therapeutic options suggested have been found to be ineffective.

Reading

Jo HE, Randhawa S, Corte TJ, et al. Idiopathic pulmonary fibrosis and the elderly: Diagnosis and management considerations. *Drugs Aging* 2016; 33: 321–334.

73 Correct Answer: B

Explanation: It is estimated that around half of people living with HIV in the developed world are now aged over 50. Many of these people became infected at a younger age, but around a sixth of new infections occur in people aged over 50. Care is made more complex by the existence of comorbidities and polypharmacy. Drug resistance and adverse effects become more likely after exposure for a long period. There is a tendency to develop comorbidities at younger ages than do people without HIV infection. Higher viral loads and lower cluster of differentiation 4 (CD4) counts are independently associated with an increased risk for cardiac ischemia. Older antiretroviral drugs were associated with an increased risk of developing diabetes. Frailty occurs at a younger age in people living with HIV. Osteoporosis is more common in people on antiretroviral drugs (estimated twofold fracture risk increase compared to age-matched controls), and bisphosphonate drugs are probably helpful in selected people. There is also an associated increased risk of falls. Neurocognitive impairment is also associated with HIV infection. The most severe form is HIV-related dementia, but more common is 'HIV Associated Neurocognitive Disorder' causing subtler symptoms. This typically affects attention, working memory, executive function and processing speed rather than impairments in long-term memory or language ability. It may affect adherence to medications.

Reading

McMillan JM, Krentz H, Gill MJ, et al. Managing HIV infection in patients older than 50 years. *CMAJ* 2018; 190: E1253–E1258.

74 Correct Answer: A

Explanation: Rapid eye movement sleep behaviour disorder (RBD) is a complex motor disorder due to dream enactment during REM sleep. It occurs more commonly in people with synucleinopathies (i.e. Parkinson's disease, dementia with Lewy bodies or multiple system atrophy) but may be idiopathic. It can present years before a neurodegenerative condition is diagnosed. Sometimes it is necessary to move the mattress onto the floor and place padding on nearby furniture to reduce the risk of injury. Some medications (e.g. antidepressants and cholinesterase inhibitors) may exacerbate symptoms, and dose reduction or discontinuation can be considered. Clonazepam or melatonin may be tried for symptom relief, including reducing the risk of injury. Both may cause daytime sleepiness. Clonazepam has a greater risk of worsening any underlying cognitive impairment. Midodrine, an alpha agonist, is sometimes used to treat orthostatic hypotension. Modafinil is a centrally acting stimulant drug that sometimes helps

with daytime sleepiness (N.B. long list of potential side effects). A rotigotine patch is sometimes used to treat nocturnal akinesia. Quetiapine is sometimes used to manage hallucinations and/or delusions in people with Parkinson's disease who do not have cognitive impairment. Such symptoms would only usually be treated if causing distress to the patient, and reducing the dose of dopaminergic medications should be considered first.

Reading

National Institute for Health and Care Excellence. Parkinson's disease in adults. 2017. www.nice.org.uk/guidance/ng71.
St Louis EK, Boeve AR, Boeve BF. REM sleep behavior disorder in Parkinson's disease and other synucleinopathies. *Movement Disorders* 2017; 32: 645–658.

75 Correct Answer: E

Explanation: Polymyalgia rheumatica (PMR) and giant cell arteritis (GCA) are related inflammatory conditions that occur almost exclusively in older people (typical diagnostic criteria of age >50 and ESR >50). Around half of people with GCA have features of PMR at diagnosis, and around 20% of people with untreated PMR will develop features of GCA. GCA can occur in cranial (C-GCA) or large vessel (LV-GCA, i.e. extracranial) subtypes. C-GCA can present with headache (67%), jaw claudication (50%), tongue pain and visual symptoms or loss (25%). Possible visual symptoms include amaurosis fugax and diplopia. If visual loss occurs then it is permanent, and unilateral blindness has a high risk of becoming bilateral after a few days if untreated. Brain or tongue infarcts are possible but uncommon. Constitutional symptoms may be present, e.g. fever, malaise, anorexia and weight loss. LV-GCA can present as pyrexia of unknown origin, limb claudication or chest/back pain (aortitis). Temporal artery ultrasound is useful in the diagnosis of C-GCA, and MRI scanning can be used for detecting aortitis in LV-GCA. PMR causes proximal pain and morning stiffness. It can also be associated with peripheral arthritis and oedema. Oral prednisolone 40–60 mg daily is typically used for the initial treatment of GCA and 15 mg daily for PMR.

Reading

Dejaco C, Duftner C, Buttgereit F, et al. The spectrum of giant cell arteritis and polymyalgia rheumatica: Revisiting the concept of the disease. *Rheumatology* 2017; 56: 506–515.

76 Correct Answer: A

Explanation: Anticoagulation following a confirmed deep vein thrombosis (DVT) or PE is recommended for at least three months. A three- to six-month duration is recommended in people with active cancer. This man has had a provoked DVT with an uncomplicated clinical course. He has no other indication to continue anticoagulation. A longer duration of anticoagulation may be appropriate if he had had an unprovoked DVT, also considering any risk of bleeding complications.

Reading

National Institute for Health and Care Excellence. Venous thromboembolic diseases: Diagnosis, management and thrombophilia testing. 2020. www. nice.org.uk/guidance/ng158.

77 Correct Answer: D

Explanation: Non-pharmacological approaches, including speech and language therapy techniques, should be offered first for people with Parkinson's disease who experience problems with speech, swallowing or saliva control. Glycopyrronium

bromide is the second option, followed by referral for botulinum toxin A injections if ineffective. Other anticholinergic medications have a greater risk of causing side effects. Topical atropine may be preferable to a systemic medication.

Reading

National Institute for Health and Care Excellence. Parkinson's disease in adults. 2017. www.nice.org. uk/guidance/ng71.

78 Correct Answer: C

Comorbidities associated with an increased risk of AAA:

- COPD
- Coronary, cerebrovascular or peripheral arterial disease
- Family history of AAA
- Hyperlipidaemia
- Hypertension
- Current or ex-smoker
- Cholecystolithiasis or diverticulosis

Reading

Müller V, Miszczuk M, Althoff CE, et al. Comorbidities associated with large abdominal aortic aneurysms. *Aorta (Stamford)* 2019; 7 (4): 108–114.
National Institute for Health and Care Excellence. Abdominal aortic aneurysm: Diagnosis and management. 2020. www.nice.org.uk/guidance/ng156.

79 Correct Answer: E

Explanation: Dopamine agonists are likely to have the biggest effect on improving duration of off time but with a higher risk of causing hallucinations than MAO-B inhibitors (e.g. rasagiline) or COMT inhibitors (e.g. entacapone). Although amantadine is sometimes used in motor fluctuations, the evidence base for both its beneficial and adverse effects is lacking. Non-ergot-derived dopamine agonists (e.g. ropinirole) are used in preference to ergot-derived ones (e.g. cabergoline) due to the risk of additional side effects with this type of medication, which also necessitates monitoring (i.e. risk of fibrosis mainly affecting the heart and lungs). A protein redistribution diet, where most of the daily protein is taken in the last meal of the day, may help with motor fluctuations for people who are taking levodopa (through improved drug absorption from the bowel).

Reading

National Institute for Health and Care Excellence. Parkinson's disease in adults. 2017. www.nice.org.uk/guidance/ng71.

80 Correct Answer: C

Explanation: Testing for rheumatoid factor is advised in all people with suspected rheumatoid arthritis and clinical evidence of synovitis. Anti-cyclic citrullinated peptide (CCP) antibodies might be tested if rheumatoid factor is negative, X-rays of the hands and feet are recommended in people with persistent synovitis and both are usually performed once a diagnosis has been established if not done already.

Reading

National Institute for Health and Care Excellence. Rheumatoid arthritis in adults: Management. 2018. www.nice.org.uk/guidance/ng100.

81 Correct Answer: A

Explanation: There is some evidence to support the efficacy of topical NSAIDs over placebo, especially topical diclofenac for osteoarthritis pain. Lidocaine patches may be effective for post-herpetic neuralgia, but there is no reliable evidence outside of this indication. A 12-month study did not find any analgesic superiority of opioids compared to non-opioids for musculoskeletal pain, and the incidence of adverse effects was higher. Gabapentin and pregabalin are options for the management of neuropathic pain only. There is some evidence that duloxetine may be useful for chronic low back pain, whereas the same is not true for tricyclic antidepressants.

Reading

Scottish Intercollegiate Guidelines Network. Management of chronic pain. Guideline 136, 2019. www.sign.ac.uk/media/1108/sign136_2019.pdf.

82 Correct Answer: C

Explanation: Over 50% of new diagnoses are due to heart failure with a preserved ejection fraction. The prognoses of systolic and diastolic heart failure are similar. One-year mortality is around 20% and five-year mortality around 50% in this age group. The age-adjusted incidence of heart failure has fallen over recent years. One of the factors impairing diastolic relaxation in older people is a prolonged period of cardiac contraction, probably due to increased cardiac stiffness and impaired calcium release and reuptake into the sarcoplasmic reticulum.

Reading

Dharmarajan K, Rich MW. Epidemiology, pathophysiology, and prognosis of heart failure in older adults. *Heart Fail Clin* 2017; 3: 381–387.

83 Correct Answer: A

Explanation: A conservative management plan for older people with end-stage renal disease in the presence of multiple comorbidities can be reasonable. In this group, survival rates compared to renal replacement therapy are similar. They are also more likely to spend less time in hospital and to die in their own home.

Time spent travelling to the unit and receiving dialysis three times a week can negatively impact quality of life. Dialysis is usually commenced when the symptoms of uraemia develop, and the control of these is likely to be its greatest benefit. More than 20% of people receiving dialysis in Europe are aged 75 or over.

Reading

Segall L, Nistor I, van Biesen W, et al. Dialysis modality choice in elderly patients with end-stage renal disease: A narrative review of the available evidence. *Nephrol Dial Transplant* 2017; 32: 41–49.

84 Correct Answer: B

Explanation: Glomerulosclerosis leading to nephron loss is the key pathological process resulting in declining renal function in older age. It is estimated that around half of people aged over 70 have an eGFR below 60, and many do not have an underlying diagnosable renal disease.

Compared to younger people, arteriovenous fistula formation takes long to mature and has a lower success rate. Older people are more prone to haemodialysis-related complications, including hypotension, infection and gastrointestinal bleeding. Peritoneal dialysis avoids the need to attend a dialysis centre three times a week or the need for vascular access (currently <25% of dialysis). Physical and cognitive functional impairment often lead to haemodialysis being chosen over peritoneal dialysis (i.e. less commonly used in people aged over 75). There probably is a small survival advantage with haemodialysis. Quality of life seems to be similar for peritoneal and haemodialysis.

Reading

Glassock RJ, Rule AD. Aging and the kidneys: Anatomy, physiology and consequences for defining chronic kidney disease. *Nephron* 2016; 134: 25–29.

Segall L, Nistor I, van Biesen W, et al. Dialysis modality choice in elderly patients with end-stage renal disease: A narrative review of the available evidence. *Nephrol Dial Transplant* 2017; 32: 41–49.

85 Correct Answer: D

Explanation: Hepatitis C is an RNA virus (HCV). Both acute and chronic infections are usually asymptomatic. Chronic infection is associated with cirrhosis and hepatocellular carcinoma (HCC). A small proportion of the chronically infected develop cryoglobulinemia, glomerulonephritis, vitiligo or lymphoma. Approximately 20% of people with chronic infection develop cirrhosis over 20 years. These people have around a 4% annual risk of developing HCC and around 25 % will develop liver failure. 90% of HCC develops in people with cirrhosis. Six-monthly ultrasound screening is recommended for people with cirrhosis. HCV has an estimated global prevalence of 1% and is the most common reason for liver transplant worldwide. Many people are unaware of their infection status and present with HCC or liver failure (e.g. gastrointestinal bleeding secondary to varices, ascites or hepatic encephalopathy). HCV treatment has developed over the past decade. Anti-viral regimens lead to a sustained virological response in most people with HCV-related liver cirrhosis.

Hepatitis B is a double stranded DNA virus (HBV). Acute HBV is usually mild and self-limiting. Liver blood test abnormalities can be cholestatic in nature. Treatment of chronic HBV aims to suppress viral replication with nucleoside analogues and thus reduce the risk of developing cirrhosis and hepatocellular carcinoma. The drugs need to be taken for the long term but have a reasonable side effect profile. Interferon therapy can lead to a cure in up to 30% of patients, but probably only a smaller proportion of older people will be cured and its use is associated with significant adverse effects.

Reading

Kemp L, Clare KE, Brennan PN, et al. New horizons in hepatitis B and C in the older adult. *Age Ageing* 2019; 48: 32–37.

86 Correct Answer: A

Explanation: Autoimmune hepatitis (AIH) lacks a specific diagnostic marker but is associated with positive anti-nuclear antibody (ANA), anti-smooth muscle antibody and hypergammaglobulinaemia. Around 20% of adult-onset AIH occurs in people aged over 60, with women three times more likely to be affected. Suspect AIH in people with acute or chronically elevated hepatic transaminases. Older people are more likely to present with cirrhosis than younger people are. There is range of possible presentations from acute liver failure to chronic fatigue. It is associated with other autoimmune diseases, including coeliac disease and rheumatoid arthritis. Treatment may not be necessary for asymptomatic or mild disease. When required, steroids are usually effective (typically started at 60 mg daily). Long-term azathioprine may be required to retain remission.

Drug-induced liver injury can mimic AIH. Possible causes include nitrofurantoin, methyldopa, atorvastatin and diclofenac. There may be associated rash, fever or eosinophilia. The abnormalities should resolve on drug discontinuation. In this woman, the likely diagnosis is AIH or drug-induced liver injury. The mild nature of her symptoms suggests that initial immunosuppressive treatment is not indicated. A reasonable first step would be to discontinue the diclofenac and see if the blood test abnormalities resolve.

Reading

Rizvi S, Gawrieh S. Autoimmune hepatitis in the elderly: Diagnosis and pharmacologic management. *Drugs Aging* 2018; 35: 589–602.

87 Correct Answer: D

Explanation: Primary chronic constipation has been classified into subtypes but with some overlap between them.

- Constipation-predominant irritable bowel syndrome—defined by the Rome III criteria and characterised by abdominal pain or discomfort associated with infrequent or difficult defaecation.
- Dyssynergic defaecation—impaired coordination of the abdominal and anorectal muscles, leading to difficulty with stool evacuation. This type of constipation may be improved by biofeedback therapy.
- Slow-transit constipation—delayed transit of stool due to an underlying gut myopathy or neuropathy.

Reading

Rao SSC, Rattanakovit K, Patcharatrakul T. Diagnosis and management of chronic constipation in adults. *Nature Rev Gastroenterol Hepatol* 2016; 13: 295–305.

88 Correct Answer: A

Explanation: Bullous pemphigoid is the most common autoimmune subepidermal blistering skin disease. It involves antibodies to components of hemidesmosomes (which promote skin adhesion). It most commonly affects older people with an average age of onset above 75 years, and women are more often affected than men are. There may be a prodromal, non-bullous phase with mild to severe pruritus and/or eczematous lesions for weeks to months. The classic feature is a generalised pruritic bullous skin eruption, with tense blisters 1 to 4 cm in diameter that are most commonly found on the flexor aspects of the limbs and over the abdomen. They can also affect the oral mucosa. There appears to be an association with neurodegenerative and cerebrovascular diseases. The diagnosis is confirmed by direct immunofluorescence microscopy. Treatment is with immunosuppressive therapies.

Reading

Bernard P, Antonicelli F. Bullous pemphigoid: A review of its diagnosis, associations and treatment. *Am J Clin Dermatol* 2017; 18: 513–528.

89 Correct Answer: E

Explanation: A calcium channel blocker is usually offered first line for people aged over 55 who do not have diabetes unless there is known intolerance, the patient develops oedema or if there is clinical evidence of heart failure. In such situations, a thiazide-like diuretic (e.g. indapamide) is more appropriate. ACEi/ARB are preferred when diabetes is present (if black African or African-Caribbean family origin then consider ARB preferentially). The next step is to add in whichever of ACEi/ARB, thiazide or CCB the patient is not currently taking until prescribed all three (or not tolerated/indicated). Consider adherence if blood pressure remains poorly controlled despite being prescribed several drugs. Ongoing poor control is classified as resistant hypertension. Ambulatory BP monitoring is recommended, and check adherence. Adding spironolactone is recommended if serum potassium is 4.5 mmol/L or less, whereas an alpha or beta blocker can be added if potassium >4.5.

Reading

National Institute for Health and Care Excellence. Hypertension in adults: Diagnosis and management. Guideline 136, 2019. www.nice.org.uk/guidance/ng136.

90 Correct Answer: E

Explanation: Benign prostatic hyperplasia is progressive prostate enlargement due to non-malignant proliferation of smooth muscle and epithelial cells. The resulting symptoms include nocturia, urgency, frequency, straining, poor flow rate and eventual urinary retention. Around 80% of men aged 70 experience lower urinary tract symptoms. Alpha-adrenergic antagonists relax the smooth muscle of the prostate and bladder neck to relieve bladder outlet obstruction. Tamsulosin is a selective alpha-1a antagonist and may have a lower risk of orthostatic hypotension than non-selective drugs (e.g. doxazosin). Common side effects are orthostatic hypotension, retrograde ejaculation and rhinitis. 5-alpha reductase inhibitors block the conversion of testosterone to dihydrotestosterone, which leads to reduced prostate size over time (e.g. finasteride or dutasteride). Possible side effects include gynaecomastia, impotence and loss of libido. There may also be an association with the development of depression. The standard surgical treatment is transurethral resection of the prostate (TURP). Newer, minimally invasive surgical procedures are being developed. These include prostatic stenting, localised tissue ablation and prostatic artery embolisation.

Reading

Bortnick E, Brown C, Simma-Chiang V, et al. Modern best practice in the management of benign prostatic hyperplasia in the elderly. *Ther Adv Urol* 2020; 12: 1–11.

91 Correct Answer: A

Explanation: Dapagliflozin is a sodium-glucose cotransporter 2 (SGLT2) inhibitor. When compared to placebo in people with heart failure with a reduced ejection fraction, both with and without diabetes, there was a lower rate of worsening heart failure or cardiovascular death.

Reading

McMurray JJV, Solomon SD, Inzucchi SE, et al. Dapagliflozin in patients with heart failure and reduced ejection fraction. *N Engl J Med* 2019; 381: 1995–2008.

92 Correct Answer: D

Explanation: Paget's disease is a disorder of bone remodelling that predominantly affects the pelvis, spine, femur, tibia and skull. It is more common in older age, males and those of white ethnicity. Sometimes there is a family history with an autosomal dominant pattern of inheritance. There is also a rôle for environmental factors. The prevalence has fallen in recent years. Most cases are asymptomatic. Bone pain is the most common presenting symptom. Bone deformities and pathological fractures (most commonly femur or tibia) are possible presentations. There is an associated higher incidence of osteoarthritis. The disorganised formation of enlarged bones can lead to hearing loss, obstructive hydrocephalus, spinal canal stenosis and paraplegia. The more vascular bone created is prone to haemorrhage during orthopaedic surgery. Osteosarcoma is a rare complication. Serum alkaline phosphatase is usually elevated.

X-ray features:

- Osteolytic areas
- Cortical and trabecular thickening
- Loss of distinction between cortex and medulla
- Osteosclerosis
- Bone expansion and deformity

Radionucleotide bone scanning can be used to outline the full extent of bone involvement.

Bisphosphonates reduce bone pain but not the incidence of pathological fractures. Calcitonin may have a rôle in people with neurological symptoms.

Reading

Ralston SH, Corral-Gudino L, Cooper C, et al. Diagnosis and management of Paget's disease of bone in adults: A clinical guideline. *J Bone Mineral Res* 2019; 34: 579–604.

93 Correct Answer: A

Explanation: The 'sick euthyroid syndrome' (or 'non-thyroidal illness syndrome') occurs in a large proportion of hospitalised patients and comprises a variety of alterations in the hypothalamus-pituitary-thyroid axis that are observed during illness. Sick euthyroid syndrome refers to changes in serum thyroid hormone and TSH levels that occur in patients with a variety of non-thyroidal illnesses, including infections, malignancies, inflammatory conditions, myocardial infarction, surgery, trauma and starvation. These abnormal thyroid function tests are not due to dysfunction of the hypothalamic-pituitary-thyroid axis.

Reading

Arnold A. Primary hyperparathyroidism: Molecular genetic insights and clinical implications. Presented at Society for Endocrinology BES 2017, Harrogate, UK. Endocrine Abstracts 50 PL1.

94 Correct Answer: D

Explanation: The diagnosis is non-alcoholic fatty liver disease (NAFLD). As the rate of obesity rises, NAFLD has become the most common cause of liver dysfunction worldwide. This man has raised liver function tests (LFTs). He is tanned, which is consistent with a clinical diagnosis of haemochromatosis, but the tan probably comes from living in Mexico. Gallstones would usually cause colicky abdominal pain rather than isolated raised LFTs. Wilson's disease occurs in young adults. Of NAFLD and AFLD, both raise LFTs and could be the cause, but NAFLD tends to raise alanine aminotransferase (ALT) more than aspartate transaminase (AST). There is a strong link between NAFLD and type 2 diabetes, even beyond adiposity. Male sex and a family history of type 2 diabetes are also associated with a greater risk of NAFLD at any given body mass index.

Reading

Sattar N, Forrest E, Preiss D. Non-alcoholic fatty liver disease. *BMJ* 2014; 349: g4596.

95 Correct Answer: A

Explanation: This man does have metastatic deposits in both adrenal glands which can impair function and cause Addison's disease. Furthermore, he has hyponatraemia, hyperkalaemia and hyperpigmentation, all of which are features seen in Addison's disease. Metastases to the adrenal glands are a frequent finding in patients with advanced malignancies like lung, breast, gastric and colorectal cancer, melanoma and non-Hodgkin's lymphoma. This occurs likely due to their rich sinusoidal supply. In addition to adrenal insufficiency that develops owing to replacement of both glands by metastases, other causes of adrenal insufficiency in cancer patients include haemorrhagic necrosis of adrenals in the context of metastatic infiltration and impaired adrenal synthesis in patients being treated with some anti-cancer drugs. Adrenal insufficiency may have an acute or a chronic presentation. Acute adrenal insufficiency known as adrenal crisis or Addisonian crisis is a life-threatening medical emergency, which presents typically with circulatory collapse. It may be uncovered or precipitated by underlying stressors such as infections, trauma, surgery and other intercurrent illnesses. SIADH and PPIs can cause hyponatraemia but not cardiovascular collapse. This is not 'progressive dwindling', a term relating to a progressive decline due to a long-term condition such as frailty or dementia.

Reading

Carvalho F, Louro F, Zakout R. Adrenal insufficiency in metastatic lung cancer. *World J Oncol* 2015; 6 (3): 375–377.

96 Correct Answer: E

Explanation: An underlying pleural pathology should be strongly suspected in the case of thickened pleura, restrictive lung function and non-specific constitutional symptoms. The bilateral pleural effusions do not appear to be causing respiratory compromise, and hence a chest drain is not indicated. In the absence of parenchymal lesions to target for tissue diagnosis, video-assisted thoracoscopic biopsy (VATS) is appropriate to distinguish a cause of pleural thickening, such as organised empyema or mesothelioma, and also to obtain tissue to differentiate mesothelioma from other primary or metastatic cancers. VATS is optimally performed with a small amount of pleural fluid in situ. Biopsies for interstitial lung disease have successfully been accomplished via VATS with a lower morbidity, less pain and a shorter hospital stay in comparison with traditional open accesses. Hypersensitivity pneumonitis should also be considered because presentations with weight loss, dyspnoea and chest tightness can be similar to pleural pathology. Bronchoalveolar lavage (BAL) would be indicated if extrinsic allergic alveolitis is a significant differential, but the lack of reticulonodular changes on chest radiograph and fibrotic changes on CT make hypersensitivity pneumonitis less likely. It is worth noting that only 20% of mesothelioma patients present with radiographic changes consistent with asbestosis, although the majority present with pleural abnormalities.

Reading

Ambrogi V, Mineo TC. VATS biopsy for undetermined interstitial lung disease under non-general anesthesia: Comparison between uniportal approach under intercostal block vs. three-ports in epidural anesthesia. *J Thorac Dis* 2014; 6 (7): 888–895.

97 Correct Answer: D

Explanation: The 2018 NICE guidelines on COPD clearly define which patients should be assessed for and offered long-term oxygen therapy (LTOT). Patients who receive LTOT should breathe supplementary oxygen for at least 15 hours a day. Patients who develop a respiratory acidosis and/or a rise in $PaCO_2$ of >1 kPa (7.5 mmHg) during an LTOT assessment may have clinically unstable disease. These patients should undergo further medical optimisation and be reassessed after four weeks. The aterial blood gas (ABG) on air meets the criteria for LTOT, as the PaO_2 is <7.3 kPa. In this scenario, after a one-hour trial of low-flow oxygen, the patient's symptoms have improved, and his PaO2 has significantly improved. However, his PCO_2 has significantly increased resulting in a respiratory acidosis.

Reading

British Thoracic Society Home Oxygen Guideline Development Group. British thoracic society guidelines for home oxygen use in adults. *Thorax* 2015; 70 (Suppl 1): i1–i43.

98 Correct Answer: B

Explanation: This is a difficult question requiring recognition of a high-pressure headache, left optic atrophy and contralateral swollen disc secondary to papilloedema. The combination of an ipsilateral optic atrophy and contralateral papilloedema is an examination favourite: Foster-Kennedy syndrome, typically caused often by an anterior cranial fossa meningioma (e.g. frontal lobe, olfactory groove, sphenoid wing), compresses on the ipsilateral optic nerve and olfactory nerve while increasing intracranial pressure for the contralateral optic nerve sheath. Idiopathic intracranial hypertension may present asymmetrically but typically produces bilateral disc swelling. It is conceivable the patient has multiple sclerosis with optic atrophy secondary to left optic neuritis, but it is unlikely in this demographic. Frontotemporal dementia may explain the behavioural and personality changes but does not account for visual symptoms. Age-related macular degeneration can mimic papillitis on fundoscopy, with deposition of Drusen making the optic disc *look* swollen. However, the fundoscopy appearance of this patient in this question is very different.

Reading

Sadun AA, Wang MY. Chapter 5, Abnormalities of the optic disc. In *Handbook of Clinical Neurology*, vol 102 (2011, pp. 2–524), Neuro-ophthalmology. Eds. Kennard C, Leigh RJ. pp. 117–157. Amsterdam, The Netherlands: Elsevier.

99 Correct Answer: E

Explanation: Chronic bacterial prostatitis/chronic pelvic pain syndrome (CBP/CPPS) is a syndrome where an infective agent is absent, and the disease is led by chronic pelvic pain symptoms and voiding symptoms in the absence of urinary tract infection. Patients with CBP/CPPS should be managed according to their individual symptom pattern—no single management pathway is suitable for all patients with these conditions. Most patients with CBP/CPPS do not have an infection, and repeated use of antibiotics such as quinolones should be avoided where no obvious benefit from infection control is evident or cultures do not support an infective aetiology. Early use of anti-neuropathic pain medication should be considered for all CBP and CP/CPPS patients refractory to initial treatments. If neuropathic pain is suspected, ensure a quick referral to the multidisciplinary team (MDT), which includes pain specialists. According to current guidelines, neuropathic pain should be explained to the patient; the management should then include stopping simple analgesics and NSAIDs, unless nociceptive/inflammatory route is suspected, and the initiation of neuropathic pain management according to NICE CG173.

Reading

NICE. CG73. Neuropathic pain in adults: Pharmacological management in non-specialist settings. www.nice.org.uk/guidance/cg173.

Rees J, Abrahams M, Doble A, Cooper A. Prostatitis Expert Reading Group (PERG). Diagnosis and treatment of chronic bacterial prostatitis and chronic prostatitis/chronic pelvic pain syndrome: A consensus guideline. *BJU Int* 2015; 116 (4): 509–525.

100 Correct Answer: D

Explanation: Although permethrin 5% cream is technically off-label for the treatment of crusted scabies, it is a critical component of the first-line regimen. It should be applied daily for seven days and then twice weekly until symptoms have resolved. When patients are unable to tolerate permethrin, second-line topical agents include benzoyl benzoate, sulphur, crotamiton and malathion.

Reading

Raffi J, Suresh R, Butler DC. Review of scabies in the elderly. *Dermatol Ther (Heidelb)* December 2019; 9 (4): 623–630.

101 Correct Answer: A

Explanation: Clause 1.1.8 of the NICE guidance.

Reading

NICE guideline. Cellulitis and erysipelas: Antimicrobial prescribing. September 2019. www.nice.org.uk/guidance/ng141.

102 Correct Answer: B

Explanation: Iron deficiency anaemia is a 'red flag sign' and needs to be managed accordingly. A good history and examination, followed by investigation with haematinics, iron levels, blood film and screening for specific conditions, are required. If a patient presents with a microcytic anaemia and low ferritin, the next reasonable step is to exclude coeliac disease. In this case coeliac has successfully been excluded. The patient is premenopausal with no actual upper GI symptoms; the next step as per British Society of Gastroenterology guidance is gastroscopy and colonoscopy.

Reading

Goddard AF, James MW, McIntyre AS, et al. Guidelines for the management of iron deficiency Anaemia. *Gut* 2011; 60: 1309–1316.

4

Cognitive Impairment
(Delirium and Dementia)

The overall learning objective of this chapter is for the reader to understand the definition of cognitive impairment, its presentation and its significance.

Delirium

LEARNING OBJECTIVE:

To be able to recognise, diagnose and manage a state of delirium presenting both acutely or subacutely in patients in hospital, in the community and in other settings.

- Biological substrates involved in delirium.
- Diagnostic criteria for delirium.
- Recognition of the major types and subtypes of delirium in acute and subacute illness states.
- Standardised measures of assessing cognitive status in delirious states.
- Relationship of delirium with dementia syndromes. ˌ
- Severity indices in delirium.

- Risk factors (including anticholinergic burden) and precipitating factors.
- Main outcomes observed, and recognition of patients who require follow-up.
- Multicomponent non-pharmacological interventions.
- The possible utility of pharmacological interventions.
- Life history of a delirium episode and afterwards.
- Rôle of drugs when other measures fail, and safe dosage.

Dementia

LEARNING OBJECTIVE:

To be able to assess and manage patients who present with dementia and also to assess and manage patients with dementia who present with other illnesses.

- Biological substrates involved in dementia.
- Assessment of cognition (including acute, chronic and rapidly deteriorating).
- Diagnosis of dementia (Alzheimer's disease, vascular dementia, mixed dementia, dementia with Lewy bodies, Parkinsonian syndromes).
- Differential diagnosis of dementia (e.g. depression, dysphasia, stroke).
- Equality and diversity considerations, including in younger people with dementia, people with intellectual disabilities and people from minority ethnic groups.
- Legal aspects of capacity and consent.
- Proportionate investigation of patients presenting with dementia, including cerebrospinal fluid, neuroimaging and neuropsychological assessment.
- Communication of diagnosis, prognosis and information about relevant support and treatment options to people with dementia and their carers.
- Personalised care and support plans, including assistive technology, extra-care housing, domiciliary care.
- The impact of dementia on the assessment and management of other illnesses.
- The impact of dementia on rehabilitation, e.g. in stroke care.
- Mechanisms of action of cognitive enhancers in dementia.
- Effect of drug treatments for dementia on other illnesses.
- Assessment of behavioural and psychological symptoms associated with dementia.
- Adverse effects of common drug treatments in dementia.
- The importance of a multidisciplinary approach to dementia.
- Effect of treatment of other illnesses on dementia.

- Working with colleagues to optimise management of people with cognitive impairment and other comorbidities.
- Physical assessment of people with cognitive impairment, including in the presence of an intellectual disability.
- Differential diagnosis of cognitive decline in people with pre-existing intellectual disability.
- Atypical presentations of dementia in people with pre-existing intellectual disability.
- Assessment scales useful to measure cognitive status in people with pre-existing intellectual disability.
- Common comorbidities that might affect management of dementia in people with pre-existing intellectual disability.
- Specialist services available for people with pre-existing intellectual disability.

Questions

Question 103

A right-handed 72-year-old female pianist first noticed a few years ago a slight shaking of the left-hand side of her body when stretching her hand to reach for something off a kitchen shelf. She then noticed difficulty in finding the right words, and her husband noticed recently that she has been blinking less frequently. Her main worries are that she has been forgetting things more often of late and whether her symptoms might progress sufficiently so as to impede her playing the piano. Examination revealed myoclonus of the outstretched left hand, and a left-limb dystonia. There was no tremor. Some postural instability was found.

What is the most likely diagnosis?

TABLE 4.1

Investigations.

MRI	Frontotemporal atrophy, more severe changes to the left
Cognitive neuropsychology	Global cognitive deterioration, but with a particularly marked dysexecutive syndrome

A. behavioural variant frontotemporal dementia

B. corticobasal syndrome

C. Creutzfeld-Jacob disease

D. dementia of the Alzheimer type

E. primary progressive aphasia

Question 104

A 72-year-old man presents with his wife to the memory clinic. His wife remarks on a change in behaviour, which first was striking in a number of socially inappropriate remarks to longstanding friends. He did not think anything was 'wrong' with him, but the accountancy firm for which he worked urged him to take early retirement a few years ago. Since retirement, he has stayed in bed all the time, such that it requires a huge amount of effort to get him motivated enough even to take a meal.

What is the most likely diagnosis?

TABLE 4.2

Investigations.

MRI	Mild bilateral frontal atrophy, more marked on the right
Cognitive neuropsychology	Very mild impairment in tests sensitive to frontal lobe function

A. behavioural variant frontotemporal dementia

B. corticobasal syndrome

C. Creutzfeld-Jacob disease

D. dementia of the Alzheimer type

E. primary progressive aphasia

Question 105

Some medications for dementia might be of especial interest to an anaesthetist arranging a general anaesthetic in a surgical operation. Which of the following scenarios might cause the most concern?

A. an emergency situation, but the anaesthetist is aware of possible drug-drug interactions

B. current use of *gingko biloba*

C. donepezil discontinued four weeks ago

D. galantamine discontinued two days ago

E. rivastigmine discontinued two days ago

Question 106

Which of the following is an activity of daily living, rather than an instrumental activity of daily living?

A. an individual's ability to manage finances

B. an individual's ability to prepare food

C. an individual's ability to shop for groceries

D. an individual's ability to use the telephone

E. an individual's ability to use the toilet

Question 107

The Montreal Cognitive Assessment (MoCA) is a widely used test of cognitive function. In the MoCA, a patient is asked to name as many words as possible beginning with the letter F. In which section of the MoCA would this instruction be given?

A. attention

B. language

C. memory

D. naming

E. visuospatial/executive function

Question 108

Getting information and support when needed from people working in health and social care can make a real difference. Which of the following statements about diagnosis and post-diagnostic support is true for dementia in England?

A. a minority of emergency admissions to hospital, in people over the age of 75, were assessed for dementia in April 2019

B. the National Institute for Health and Care Excellence quality standard on dementia states that people with dementia should be given the opportunity to discuss advance care planning at diagnosis and at each health and social care review

C. primary care general practitioner data shows that, in 2018/19, a minority of people diagnosed with dementia had a face-to-face care plan review in the preceding 12 months

D. virtually all people aged 65 or older with dementia have a formal diagnosis

E. there is remarkable consistency in the estimated diagnosis rate of dementia for people aged 65 or older

Question 109

Which of the following statements is the *least* true about agitation in dementia?

A. agitation affects a minority of older medical inpatients with dementia

B. agitation can be a product of failed communication

C. agitation is likely to represent a clinically significant level of distress

D. manifestations of agitation can include pacing

E. organisational culture is relevant to the clinical management of agitation

Question 110

In neuropsychological assessment of individuals with intellectual disabilities, a battery of very simple tests covering memory, orientation, language and praxis is widely used. This battery takes about 45 minutes to administer. The majority of people with Down's syndrome can attempt most of it. It is said by the authors to be in use in over 30 intellectual disabilities services in the UK. What is it?

A. Alzheimer's Disease Assessment Scale-Cognition ('ADAS-Cog')

B. Ages and Stages Questionnaire

C. Neuropsychological Assessment of Dementia in Adults with Intellectual Disabilities

D. The Parents' Evaluation of Developmental Status Test

E. Test for severe impairment

Question 111

A previously healthy 75-year-old Chinese woman presented on the acute medical take in an unconsciousness state. The patient's family reported that she had a sudden onset of dizziness in the preceding month and recurrent attacks, but the patient did not pay attention to them. Half a month previously, her family noticed she suffered from memory disturbance, when she sometimes forgot to pull the key out of the door when leaving, forgot to close the refrigerator door and complained of money being stolen. A week before admission, the patient's symptoms slowly and gradually worsened.

TABLE 4.3

Investigations.

Laboratory haematology and biochemistry	Normal
EEG	Synchronous extensibility and high amplitude (2–2.3 Hz) of a triphasic sharp wave
CSF	14–3–3 protein detected
MRI	Minor increase in signal intensity in the bilateral parietal-occipital and frontal lobes in diffusion-weighted imaging. Cortical ribboning on FLAIR.

What is the most likely diagnosis?

A. behavioural variant frontotemporal dementia

B. corticobasal syndrome

C. Creutzfeld-Jacob disease

D. dementia of the Alzheimer type

E. primary progressive aphasia

Question 112

'Personalisation' is as a broad philosophy, which encapsulates policies not only in health, but also across public services. One of the themes is described as 'service users who are more involved in shaping the service they receive should be expected to become more active in their own service delivery'. What does this refer to?

A. advocacy

B. co-production

C. enhanced voice

D. expanded choice

E. intimate consultation

Question 113

A 72-year-old Vietnamese, retired, male chef presented with progressive speech difficulties over 18 months. There has been no change in personality or behaviour. The main problem was verbal expression with comprehension of both spoken and written language intact. His family had noticed emotional lability, which exacerbates his speech impairment. He also reported mild short-term memory loss, although this did not impact on his activities of daily living. It was previously noted that he had had intact pre-morbid language functions. Currently, he exhibits mild impairment of recall and marked visuospatial difficulties; there are, however, mild difficulties with mental calculations and mild difficulties in constructional praxis. Past medical history was unremarkable apart from hypertension. Physical examination was normal. Mini-Mental State Examination score was 22 with deficits in recall and calculation. There were no signs to suggest parietal lobe involvement.

What is the most likely diagnosis?

A. behavioural variant frontotemporal dementia

B. corticobasal syndrome

C. Creutzfeld-Jacob disease

D. dementia of the Alzheimer type

E. primary progressive aphasia

TABLE 4.4

Investigations.

Laboratory haematology and biochemistry investigations	Normal
MRI brain	Normal hippocampi
SPECT brain	Slight reduction in perfusion to the left frontal and medial frontal cortex and at the anterior temporal poles
PET brain	Marked atrophy and hypometabolism of the medial frontal lobes, including the anterior cingulate gyrus; hypometabolism of the temporal lobes and in the prefrontal cortex, but preserved activity in the anterolateral frontal cortex

Question 114

Galantamine is a drug used in the management of mild-to-moderate Alzheimer's disease.

Which of the following statements about galantamine is correct?

A. galantamine can improve the burden on carers

B. galantamine hydrobromide is a tertiary alkaloid drug

C. it is a non-allosteric modulator of nicotinic acetylcholine receptors

D. it is a reversible, competitive inhibitor of acetylcholinesterase

E. it is extensively metabolised in numerous pathways, mainly in the liver

Question 115

An 86-year-old presented to memory clinic, having been recently sacked from working as a teacher because of his 'odd' behaviour. He himself thought nothing was wrong with him, so the relevant history was actively sought by speaking with the caregiver alone. Even though forgetfulness was volunteered as the presenting complaint, careful questioning suggests that the patient's memory for everyday events is well maintained. It soon transpired that his personality had significantly changed within the last year. It turned out that the patient has said a number of things which had embarrassed other parties; he seemed to be less warm or affectionate (especially toward grandchildren and the pet cats). Within the last few months, he had recently developed new hobbies or interests, especially with a religious or spiritual bent. He did not report any incidents of 'seeing things which were not there'. On examination, he appeared impulsive and distractible.

TABLE 4.5

Investigations.

Blood tests	Normal
Brain magnetic resonance imaging (MRI)	Frontal and anterior temporal lobe atrophy, sparing of posterior cortical areas
Cognitive assessment	Deficits in executive function, requiring formulation of a strategy, response inhibition or abstraction. Test performance of memory, attention and perception in normal range

What is the most likely diagnosis?

A. dementia of Alzheimer type

B. diffuse Lewy body dementia

C. frontotemporal dementia (*behavioural variant*)

D. frontotemporal dementia (*temporal variant*)

E. posterior cortical atrophy

Question 116

An 85-year-old man presents with a 15-month history of fluctuating cognitive impairment most marked in the visuospatial domains, Parkinsonism, intermittent confusion and generalised myoclonus. His short-term memory seems very good. He was started on 62.5 mg three times daily of co-careldopa. Eye movements were normal. He has recently been reported to have unsteadiness and falls.

What is the most likely diagnosis?

A. dementia of Alzheimer type

B. diffuse Lewy body disease

C. idiopathic Parkinson's disease

D. multiple system atrophy

E. progressive supranuclear palsy

Question 117

A 74-year-old Italian-speaking woman was admitted early in the morning to the oncology unit for ongoing treatment of advanced uterine cancer, for which she had been receiving fentanyl. She had been living alone in her home but still maintaining daily activities and an active social life. Her daughter lives nearby and visits her intermittently throughout the week. Forty-eight hours after admission, the nurses reported that the admitted patient was not sleeping, restless, distressed, crying intermittently and 'shaky'. For the past several hours, she had been having frequent loose stools

TABLE 4.6

Investigations.

Urine culture	10,000 coliforms

too. In addition, the staff reported that she was talking loudly in Italian when no one was in the room. An interpreter was belatedly called, and no symptoms of urinary tract infection were reported. She, however, kept pointing to her mouth. The only intervention that seemed to help her was allowing her to drive up and down the corridors in her wheelchair. The clinical nurse specialist began to suspect pain as a possible cause of the delirium, but, prior to its onset, her pain scale was negative. The clinical nurse specialist assessed her using an observational pain scale which was positive, and pain was then confirmed through a comprehensive assessment. The admitting consultant decided to examine her mouth, and she indeed had an area of markedly inflamed gums.

She is apyrexial.

Which one of the following is the *least* likely cause of the delirium?

A. an error in medication prescribing

B. care transition

C. inadvertent cessation of fentanyl

D. language barrier

E. urinary tract infection

Question 118

An 80-year-old man presents with an abrupt change in personality and behaviour, reported by his primary carer. The National Institute for Health and Care Excellence suggests screening for possible delirium based on four risk factors. Which one of the following is *not* one of these factors?

A. age 65 or over

B. dementia

C. presentation with hip fracture

D. previous exposure to anaesthetic agents or surgical procedures

E. severity of illness

Question 119

According to the 2019 Scottish Intercollegiate Guidelines Network (SIGN) guidance, which of the following should be used for identifying patients with probable delirium in emergency department and acute hospital settings?

A. 4AT test

B. Confusion Assessment Method

C. Delirium Observation Screening Scale

D. Intensive Care Delirium Screening Checklist

E. Single Question in Delirium

Question 120

According to the 2019 Scottish Intercollegiate Guidelines Network (SIGN) guidance on delirium, which one of the following components should be considered as part of a package of care for patients at risk of developing delirium?

A. a noisy environment

B. deprescribing of pain control

C. late physiotherapy

D. maintaining optimal hydration and nutrition

E. trial without sensory aids

Question 121

The 'Delirium Index' is an instrument for the measurement of the severity of symptoms in delirium. Which of the following statements is true about it?

A. frequent, threatening hallucinations on their own will score two because of being perceptual disturbances

B. it is based on information from a family member

C. it is based on information from medication charts

D. it is based on information from nursing staff

E. the total score is the sum of seven items

Question 122

A 90-year-old Caucasian male individual awoke suddenly at about 23:00, one hour after taking a 200 mg dose of amitriptyline. His wife, who was also in the bedroom at the time, was alarmed to see the patient suddenly rise from bed and disrobe for no apparent reason. When asked what he was doing, the patient replied that he needed to get ready for work, which was bizarre, as he had retired a few years previously. Before his wife could question him, he dashed into the kitchen and began pulling out pots and pans from a bottom cabinet. He screamed, 'I can't see what I'm looking for, as it's so blurry.' Previous medications included antihistamine H_1 medications, occasional salbutamol inhalers and steroids for chronic obstructive pulmonary disease. On later examination in the accident and emergency department, he looked red, and he was found to be tachycardic, disorientated in both time and place, and to have a palpable bladder. Abnormalities in which of the following neurotransmitter systems is most likely to have contributed predominantly to the delirium?

A. acetylcholine

B. dopamine

C. GABA

D. melatonin

E. serotonin

Question 123

Haloperidol needs to be used with care, if not contraindicated, in delirium, partly because of its effect on the QT interval. The normal QT interval in men, in milliseconds (ms), has which duration?

A. 300–350 ms

B. 350–400 ms

C. 400–450 ms

D. 450–500 ms

E. 500–550 ms

Question 124

An 83-year-old man has recently been discharged from the acute medical unit for an admission due to acute loss of smell, a dry cough and shortness of breath, proven to be infection with coronavirus. He now seems to want to lie in bed. He is polite when approached, but sleepy, and he does not seem interested in eating or drinking. He looks depressed, and he has been off his food for two days. Sometimes his speech is incoherent, and he does not seem to follow what is said to him. On review by a general practitioner, his symptoms are thought to be a hypoactive delirium, rather than an ongoing infection with coronavirus.

Which of the following is true of this type of delirium?

A. it has worse outcomes than hyperactive delirium

B. it is best treated with sertraline

C. it is frequently easily identified

D. it is less common than hyperactive delirium

E. it is not associated with increased mortality

Question 125

A foundation year doctor is testing a patient whom she thinks might have delirium using the 4AT. She asks the patient, 'Please tell me the months of the year in backwards order, starting at December', and then to assist initial understanding, she provides one prompt of 'What is the month before December?'. The patient is unable to start. How much would this category, known as 'the months of the year backwards', of the 4AT score?

A. 0

B. 1

C. 2

D. 3

E. 4

Question 126

An 80-year-old man has been taking donepezil 10 mg each morning since he was diagnosed with Alzheimer's disease about three years ago. At annual review, his dementia is now moderately severe and his wife says that he is more agitated and restless, especially at night. He has no history of convulsions. What would be the most appropriate pharmacological management?

A. reduce dose of donepezil to 5 mg

B. start low dose of risperidone

C. start memantine 5 mg once daily

D. start memantine 20 mg once daily

E. take donepezil in evening, rather than in morning

Question 127

A 77-year-old woman presents with an 18-month history of forgetfulness and recently became lost on returning home. There is a longstanding history of hypertension treated with atenolol. She appears euthymic and scores 77/100 on an ACE-III test with deficits in multiple domains. She has a normal examination, except for a pulse rate of 50 and ankle oedema. What is the most appropriate next step?

A. reduce, and then stop atenolol

B. start donepezil 5 mg od

C. start donepezil 10 mg od

D. start galantamine 4 mg bd

E. start memantine 5 mg od

Question 128

A 92-year-old woman, who lives alone, is taken to her GP because her daughter is concerned that she has been deteriorating over the last few weeks. There was a concern that her flat contained a blocked flue. Her clinical condition had improved slightly over Easter while staying with family, but since returning home she has become increasingly muddled, has difficulty concentrating, feels dizzy and complains of nausea, malaise and headache. What is the most likely diagnosis?

A. anxiety and depression

B. carbon monoxide poisoning

C. hypothyroidism

D. influenza

E. medication overuse

Question 129

A 97-year-old woman with a diagnosis of Alzheimer's dementia, who is currently an inpatient on your ward, asks you to phone her father urgently and tell him that she will be late home. She was admitted following a fall in her bungalow, where she lives alone. She scored 9 out of 30 on a recent Montreal Cognitive Examination test. Which reply is most appropriate?

A. 'How old is your father?'

B. 'I can't do that because I am very busy at the moment, but can I get you a drink?'

C. 'Tell me about your father.'

D. 'Yes, I'll phone him now.'

E. 'Your father died some years ago.'

Question 130

An 85-year-old man presented with a five-day history of increasing confusion. He had been visited at home by his general practitioner (GP) and was disorientated in time, place and person. The patient gave no history of chest pain, breathlessness, urinary frequency or dysuria. He did not appear breathless or cyanosed. He denied any falls and did not appear to have any bruising. His GP had sent him to the acute medical unit for further assessment. The patient had a history of hypertension. His daily medication comprised aspirin 75 mg, bendroflumethiazide 2.5 mg od, atorvastatin 20 mg nocte and atenolol 50 mg od. On examination, his temperature was 36.9°C, his pulse was 70 beats/min and his blood pressure was 135/70 mmHg. He was clinically dehydrated. Chest examination showed scattered bi-basal crackles, with normal oxygen saturation breathing air. His neurological examination was normal. There was no evidence of loin tenderness. A diagnosis of delirium was made using the 4AT. Urinalysis was negative.

TABLE 4.7

Investigations.

White cell count	9.5×10^9/L (4.0–11.0)
Serum sodium	115 mmol/L (137–144)
Serum urea	13.0 mmol/L (2.5–7.0)

What is the most appropriate treatment of his acute confusion?

A. intravenous sodium chloride solution 0.9%

B. intravenous sodium chloride solution 3%

C. oral nitrofurantoin

D. oral trimethoprim

E. restrict fluid to 1 L/day

Question 131

A 77-year-old woman is admitted to the acute medical unit with acute confusion. Her past medical history includes a stroke eight months previously, post-stroke seizures, hypertension, osteoporosis, atrial fibrillation and weight gain. Her medications include apixaban, amlodipine, sodium valproate, paracetamol and ramipril. She denies any alcohol history. On examination her observations are normal and there is no new focal neurology.

Investigations reveal:

What is the most likely diagnosis?

A. hepatic encephalopathy

B. hypertensive encephalopathy

C. uraemic encephalopathy

D. Wernicke's encephalopathy

E. valproate encephalopathy

TABLE 4.8

Investigations.

Haemoglobin	110 g/L (130–180)
Platelet count	347 × 10⁹/L (150–400)
White cell count	10.1 × 10⁹/L (4.0–11.0)
Serum sodium	138 mmol/L (137–144)
Serum potassium	3.9 mmol/L (3.5–4.9)
Serum urea	5.2 mmol/L (2.5–7.0)
Serum creatinine	90 mmol/L (60–110)

Serum total bilirubin	6 μmol/L (1–22)
Serum alkaline phosphatase	110 U/L (45–105)
Serum alanine transferase	15 U/L (5–35)
Albumin	34 g/L (35–50)
Ammonia level	280 (elevated)
CT head	Old left middle cerebral artery infarct; no intracranial haemorrhage.

Question 132

Which of the following statements concerning neuroimaging in dementia is correct?

A. 3T MRI scanners are used most in clinical practice

B. structural imaging can reveal atrophy decades prior to the onset of symptoms in individuals with certain types of dementia

C. neuroimaging changes are rarely stated as supportive criteria for the diagnosis of neurodegenerative disease

D. weaker magnetic fields are particularly useful in identifying cerebral microbleeds

E. weaker magnetic fields are particularly useful in identifying subfields of the hippocampus

Answers for Chapter 4

103 Correct Answer: B

Explanation: The history makes corticobasal syndrome (CBS) the most likely diagnosis here. Symptoms usually begin between the ages of 50 and 70. Because signs and symptoms associated with corticobasal degeneration are frequently caused by other neurodegenerative disorders, researchers use the term 'corticobasal syndrome' to indicate the clinical diagnosis based on signs and symptoms. Visuospatial deficits are commonly reported. Typical MRI findings in CBS are asymmetric cortical atrophy, mainly frontoparietal, with the most severe changes contralateral to the more affected clinical side.

Reading

A useful webpage on the corticobasal syndrome can be found at https://rarediseases.org/rare-diseases/corticobasal-degeneration/.

Pillon B, Blin J, Vidailhet M, et al. The neuropsychological pattern of corticobasal degeneration: Comparison with progressive supranuclear palsy and Alzheimer's disease. *Neurology* August 1995; 45 (8): 1477–1483.

104 Correct Answer: A

Explanation: Patients with behavioural variant frontotemporal dementia can show a mixture of disinhibition and apathy. Apathy is characterised by loss of interest in personal affairs and responsibilities, social withdrawal and loss of awareness of personal hygiene. Disinhibition is manifested by a large amount of socially inappropriate behaviours, such as making inappropriate or insensitive remarks to others. Insight can be impaired, with either obvious denial of illness or very shallow recognition of their problem.

Reading

Sheelakumari R, Bineesh C, Varghese T, Kesavadas C, Verghese J, Mathuranath PS. Neuroanatomical correlates of apathy and disinhibition in behavioural variant frontotemporal dementia. *Brain Imaging Behav* October 2020; 14 (5): 2004–2011.

105 Correct Answer: B

Explanation: Gingko biloba is used to treat memory loss but may interfere with platelet function leading to impaired haemostasis. It is recommended that all herbal medicines such as gingko biloba are discontinued two weeks before surgery. Therefore current use of gingko biloba would be problematic. Available guidelines suggest stopping these acetylcholinesterase inhibitors before elective surgery. Both galantamine and rivastigmine have short half-lives (7–8 and 3–4 hours, respectively) and can be discontinued even the day before surgery. Donepezil has a long half-life of 70 hours and would require a washout period of 2–3 weeks. In situations where it is not practical to stop anticholinesterase therapy such as emergency surgery, the anaesthetist should be aware of the potential for interactions and consider avoiding neuromuscular blocking agents altogether.

Reading

Alcorn S, Foo I. Perioperative management of patients with dementia. *BJA Education* 2017; 17: 94–98.

106 Correct Answer: E

Explanation: When evaluating older people, it is important to assess cognitive status and determine their baseline ability to function and perform activities of daily living (ADLs). ADLs relate to personal care including bathing or showering, dressing, getting in or out of bed or a chair, using the toilet, and eating. Instrumental activities of daily living (IADLs) include the individual's ability to prepare food, manage finances, shop for groceries, do housework and use the telephone. Having a baseline for a patient's ADLs and IADLs allows the physician to recognise and act upon changes.

Reading

Gagliardi JP. Differentiating among depression, delirium, and dementia in elderly patients. *Virtual Mentor* 2008; 10 (6): 383–388.

107 Correct Answer: B

Explanation: This letter fluency task is given as part of testing language in the MoCA.

Reading

www.mocatest.org/wp-content/uploads/2015/tests-instructions/MoCA-Test-English_7_1.pdf.

108 Correct Answer: B

Explanation: The NICE quality standard on dementia states that people with dementia should be given the opportunity to discuss advance care planning at diagnosis and at each health and social care review. The other statements are false. For example, 92% of emergency admissions to hospital, in people over the age of 75, were assessed for dementia in April 2019. Primary care GP data shows that, in 2018/19, 78% of people diagnosed with dementia had a face-to-face care plan review in the preceding 12 months. Not everyone with dementia has a formal diagnosis. In March 2019, NHS Digital estimated that two thirds (68.7%) of people aged 65 or older with dementia have a formal diagnosis. Higher diagnosis rates may be due to some areas prioritising dementia diagnosis and increased awareness of the importance of making a timely diagnosis.

Reading

National Institute for Health and Care Excellence. Referral, diagnosis and care planning. www.nice.org.uk/about/what-we-do/into-practice/measuring-the-use-of-nice-guidance/impact-of-our-guidance/niceimpact-dementia/ch2-referral-diagnosis-and-care-planning.

109 Correct Answer: A

Explanation: The first statement is least true as agitation in dementia, as it is currently understood, affects over 40% of care home residents and 75% of older medical hospital inpatients with dementia. Agitation is broadly defined as restlessness, pacing, shouting, and verbal or physical aggression; it is complex and multifactorial with a range of biological, psychological and social causes. It may be a direct result of neurodegeneration, affecting brain circuits that control behaviour, and also an expression of unmet needs (e.g. pain or thirst, lack of communication or comfort), indicating emotional distress. Sometimes deemed as aggression or challenging behaviour, agitation can be difficult, harmful and exhausting for patients and carers. Organisational support and leadership are key drivers of good-quality dementia and end-of-life care in care homes and acute hospitals. Staff can report feeling stigmatised and intimidated by managers, producing further 'malignant interactions' when people are agitated.

Reading

Sampson EL, Stringer A, La Frenais F, et al. Agitation near the end of life with dementia: An ethnographic study of care. *PLoS One* 2019; 14 (10): e0224043.

110 Correct Answer: C

Explanation: The description is of the 'Neuropsychological Assessment of Dementia in Adults with Intellectual Disabilities'. Such measures should be used only for screening.

Reading

Dementia and people with intellectual disabilities: Guidance on the assessment, diagnosis, interventions and support of people with intellectual disabilities. RCPsych/BPS April 2015. www.bps.

111 Correct Answer: C

Explanation: Creutzfeldt-Jakob disease (CJD) is a rare, fatal, neurodegenerative disorder characterised by rapidly progressive dementia and neurological signs. CJD belongs to the group of transmissible spongiform encephalopathies, which share the neuropathologic triad of spongiform degeneration of the brain, neuronal death and astrocytic gliosis. There are different forms of CJD. The most common form (85%) is sporadic CJD (sCJD); the cause of the disease is unknown. The clinical diagnosis of sCJD is based on clinical signs, characteristic results on EEG and detection of the protein 14–3–3 in the CSF. Typical findings on MR imaging in sCJD are signal hyperintensity abnormalities in the cortical and deep grey matter. With the introduction of fluid-attenuated inversion recovery (FLAIR) and diffusion-weighted imaging, cortical ribbon-like high-signal intensity has increasingly been described.

Reading

Tschampa HJ, Kallenberg K, Kretzschmar HA, et al. Pattern of cortical changes in sporadic Creutzfeldt-Jakob disease. *JNR Am J Neuroradiol* 2007; 28 (6): 1114–1118.

Xu Y, Xu J, Zhang J, et al. Sporadic Creutzfeldt-Jakob disease presenting as dizziness and cognitive decline: A case report. *Medicine* (Baltimore) 2019; 98 (24): e16002.

112 Correct Answer: B

Explanation: This question concerns defining 'co-production'.

Suggested definitions are:

- *Advocacy*: professionals should act as advocates for service users, helping them to navigate through the system.
- *Co-production*: service users who are more involved in shaping the service they receive should be expected to become more active in their own service delivery.
- *Intimate consultation*: professionals work with service users to unlock their needs, preference and aspirations.
- *Enhanced voice*: articulating preference is easier for service users if they are able to make comparisons between alternatives.
- *Expanded choice*: service users are given greater choice over the way their needs might be met.

Reading

Skills for Health. Scoping for Personalisation. Final Report. 24 November 2009. www.skillsforhealth. org.uk/images/resource-section/service-area/ dementia/scoping-for-personalisation-report-ml. pdf.

113 Correct Answer: E

Explanation: The clinical vignette describes primary progressive aphasia; the neuroimaging findings are fairly typical.

Diagnostic criteria for primary progressive aphasia are:

- Gradual progression of word-finding, object-naming or word comprehension impairments.
- All limitation of daily living activities can be attributed to the language impairment, for at least two years after onset.
- Intact pre-morbid language functions.
- Absence of significant apathy, disinhibition, forgetfulness for recent events,

visuospatial impairment, visual recognition deficits or sensorimotor dysfunction within the initial two years of illness.

- Acalculia and ideomotor apraxia can be present even in the first two years.
- Other domains may become affected after the first two years, but language remains the most impaired function throughout the course of the illness and deteriorates faster than other affected domains.
- Absence of specific causes such as stroke or tumour.

Reading

Hong FS, Sinnappu RN, Lim WK. Primary progressive aphasia: A case report. *Age Ageing* 2007; 36 (6): 700–702.

Mesulam MM. Primary progressive aphasia and the language network: The 2013 H. Houston Merritt Lecture. *Neurology* 2013; 81 (5): 456–462.

114 Correct Answer: A

Explanation: Carer burden (time spent by carers supervising patients or assisting them with ADL) and caregiver distress (related to patients' behavioural symptoms) are found to be both reduced with galantamine. Galantamine has a unique, dual mode of action. It is a reversible, competitive inhibitor of acetylcholinesterase, and is the only drug actively marketed for the treatment of Alzheimer's disease with proven activity as an allosteric modulator of nicotinic acetylcholine receptors. During four large randomised, double-blind, placebo-controlled trials of up to six months duration, galantamine 16 and 24 mg/day significantly benefited cognitive and global function, ability to perform activities of daily living and behaviour, relative to placebo and baseline, for up to six months.

Reading

Lilienfeld S. Galantamine—a novel cholinergic drug with a unique dual mode of action for the treatment of patients with Alzheimer's disease. *CNS Drug Rev* 2002; 8 (2): 159–176.

115 Correct Answer: C

Explanation: The history, examination and investigation findings are typical of the behavioural variant of frontotemporal dementia (bvFTD). bvFTD is a clinical syndrome characterised by a progressive deterioration of personality, social interaction and cognition. These changes result from frontotemporal lobar degeneration associated with a range of heterogeneous pathologies. There are no objective deficits in memory, perception or language, excluding the other options.

Diagnostic criteria for probable behavioural variant frontotemporal dementia: Based on recent empirical knowledge, the International Behavioural Variant FTD Criteria Consortium (FTDC) developed revised guidelines for the diagnosis of bvFTD (international consensus criteria for behavioural variant FTD, https://www.theaftd.org/wp-content/uploads/2009/02/Table-3-International-consensus-criteria-for-behavioural-variant-FTD.pdf).

All of the following symptoms (A–C) must be present to meet criteria.

A. Meets criteria for possible bvFTD

B. Exhibits significant functional decline (by caregiver report or as evidenced by Clinical Dementia Rating Scale or Functional Activities Questionnaire scores)

C. Imaging results consistent with bvFTD (one of the following (C.1 or C.2) must be present):

   C.1. Frontal and/or anterior temporal atrophy on MRI or CT

C.2. Frontal and/or anterior temporal hypoperfusion or hypometabolism on PET or SPECT

Reading

Rahman S, Sahakian BJ, Hodges JR, et al. Specific cognitive deficits in mild frontal variant frontotemporal dementia. *Brain* 1999; 122: 1469–1493.

Rahman, S, Howard, R. *Essentials of dementia.* London: Jessica-Kingsley Publishers, 2018.

Rascovsky K, Hodges JR, Knopman D, et al. Sensitivity of revised diagnostic criteria for the behavioural variant of frontotemporal dementia. *Brain* 2011; 134: 2456–2477.

Warren JD, Rohrer JD, Rossor MN. Clinical review. Frontotemporal dementia. *BMJ* 2013; 347: f4827.

116 Correct Answer: B

Explanation: The presentation is typical of dementia with Lewy bodies. People with dementia with Lewy bodies may have:

* Hallucinations—seeing, hearing or smelling things that are not there.
* Problems with understanding, thinking, memory, judgement, confusion or sleepiness—this can change over minutes or hours.
* Slow movement, stiff limbs and tremors (uncontrollable shaking).
* Disturbed sleep, often with violent movements and shouting out.
* Fainting spells, unsteadiness and falls.

There is less short-term memory impairment so characteristic of Alzheimer's disease, and the presentation is not one of idiopathic Parkinson's disease. Eye movements, limb rigidity, hallucinations fluctuations and visuospatial impairment all point towards dementia with Lewy bodies; in contrast, early falls, frontal affect, axial rigidity and eye movement abnormalities all point to progressive supranuclear palsy.

Reading

NHS website: Dementia with Lewy bodies. www.nhs.uk/conditions/dementia-with-lewy-bodies/.

117 Correct Answer: E

Explanation: The cause of delirium is likely to be due to an acute withdrawal of fentanyl. Medication errors are common as a cause of delirium among older adults. Transitions of care, even transition from home to hospital, can increase the likelihood of errors and missing information. Current evidence appears insufficient to accurately determine if UTI and confusion are associated, with estimates varying widely. This was often attributable to poor case definitions for UTI or confusion, or inadequate control of confounding factors. A language barrier might have contributed to the delirium, as a lack of response to the patient's Italian speaking aloud could have precipitated a distressed behaviour.

Reading

Case Study: Delirium in an Older, Hospitalized Woman. https://deliriumnetwork.org/case-study-delirium-in-an-older-hospitalized-woman/.

Mayne S, Bowden A, Sundvall PD, et al. The scientific evidence for a potential link between confusion and urinary tract infection in the elderly is still confusing—a systematic literature review. *BMC Geriatr* 2019; 19 (1): 32.

118 Correct Answer: D

Explanation: These NICE recommendations were developed from studies of a wide range of clinical populations recruited from surgical, intensive care and general medical settings. It is important to recognise that delirium risk factors may differ between medical and surgical patients where the latter are exposed to iatrogenic factors such as anaesthetic agents or surgical procedures.

Reading

Ahmed S, Leurent B, Sampson EL. Risk factors for incident delirium among older people in acute hospital medical units: A systematic review and meta-analysis. *Age Ageing* 2014; 43 (3): 326–333.

119 Correct Answer: A

Explanation: Delirium is frequently missed in routine clinical care and lack of detection is associated with poor outcomes. Delirium detection should ideally be undertaken at the earliest opportunity. Numerous assessment tools have been developed to help identify probable delirium in patients in a variety of settings, which can then prompt a more accurate diagnosis and consideration of underlying causes, but the strongest evidence appears to be for the 4AT currently.

Reading

Rahman, S. *Essentials of delirium*. London: Jessica-Kingsley Publishers, 2020.
Scottish Intercollegiate Guidelines Network. Risk reduction and management of delirium. *SIGN* 157. www.sign.ac.uk/assets/sign157.pdf.
Tieges Z, Maclullich AMJ, Anand A, et al. Diagnostic accuracy of the 4AT for delirium detection in older adults: Systematic review and meta-analysis. *Age Ageing* 2020; afaa224.

120 Correct Answer: D

Explanation: According to the current SIGN guidance, the following components should be considered as part of a package of care for patients at risk of developing delirium:

- Orientation and ensuring patients have their glasses and hearing aids
- Promoting sleep hygiene
- Early mobilisation
- Pain control
- Prevention, early identification and treatment of postoperative complications
- Maintaining optimal hydration and nutrition
- Regulation of bladder and bowel function
- Provision of supplementary oxygen, if appropriate

Reading

Scottish Intercollegiate Guidelines Network. Risk reduction and management of delirium. SIGN 157. www.sign.ac.uk/assets/sign157.pdf.

121 Correct Answer: E

Explanation: The full index is here:

www.smhc.qc.ca/ignitionweb/data/ media_centre_files/510/Delirium% 20Index%20July%2027_%202011. pdf

Reading

McCusker J, Cole M, Bellavance F, et al. The reliability and validity of a new measure of severity of delirium. *Int Psychogeriatr* 1998; 10 (4): 421–433.
McCusker J, Cole M, Dendukuri N, et al. The delirium index, a measure of the severity of delirium: New findings on reliability, validity, and responsiveness. *J Am Geriatr Soc* 2004; 52 (10): 1744–1749.

122 Correct Answer: A

Explanation: The description is of a classical anticholinergic syndrome which should be readily diagnosed by the experienced clinician ('hot as a hare, red as a beet, dry as a bone, blind as a bat and mad as a hatter'). Drugs with anticholinergic properties are commonly prescribed in older persons. These drugs are associated with a wide spectrum of adverse effects including dizziness, blurred vision, urinary retention, constipation, confusion and possibly also delirium. Medications are an important risk factor for delirium and may be the sole precipitant for many cases of delirium. It is therefore sensible to conduct a drug review for patients at risk of delirium. Ideally, such a review should be informed by an evidence base that identifies those agents at highest associated risk for delirium. However, a review has found that there is a paucity of data from higher quality prospective studies for a number of classes of medication. Side effects associated with tricyclic antidepressant (TCA) therapy often leads to premature drug discontinuation. The most common side effects associated with TCAs are those related to the anticholinergic activity of these medicines.

Reading

Clegg A, Young JB. Which medications to avoid in people at risk of delirium: A systematic review. *Age Ageing* 2011; 40 (1): 23–29.

123 Correct Answer: C

Explanation: The normal QT interval is 400–450 ms in men.

Reading

Al-Khatib SM, LaPointe NM, Kramer JM, et al. What clinicians should know about the QT interval. *JAMA* 2003; 289 (16): 2120–2127.

124 Correct Answer: A

Explanation: All the other statements are false. The stem refers to *hypoactive delirium*. Current published evidence suggests that hypoactive delirium is associated with a higher risk of mortality.

Reading

Yang FM, Marcantonio ER, Inouye SK, et al. Phenomenological subtypes of delirium in older persons: Patterns, prevalence, and prognosis. *Psychosomatics* 2009; 50 (3): 248–254.
Young J, Inouye SK. Delirium in older people. *BMJ* 2007; 334 (7598): 842–846.

125 Correct Answer: C

The 4AT is a test for the rapid screening of delirium in routine clinical practice and has been shown to be a sensitive and specific method of screening for delirium in hospitalised older people. It is noted for its brevity and its ease to use.

Reading

Bellelli G, Morandi A, Davis DH, Mazzola P, Turco R, Gentile S, Ryan T, Cash H, Guerini F, Torpilliesi T, Del Santo F, Trabucchi M, Annoni G, MacLullich AM. Validation of the 4AT, a new instrument for rapid delirium screening: a study in 234 hospitalised older people. *Age Ageing* July 2014; 43 (4): 496–502.
4AT rapid clinical test for delirium. www.the4at.com (accessed 9th July 2021).

126 Correct Answer: C

Explanation: Memantine is a glutamate receptor antagonist, indicated for moderate to severe dementia in Alzheimer's disease. Starting dose of memantine is 5 mg once daily. Maintenance dose is 20 mg per day.

Reading

British National Formulary. Memantine bnf.nice.org.uk/drug/memantine-hydrochloride.html#indicationsAndDoses.

127 Correct Answer: A

Explanation: ACE-III is a detailed test, scored out of 100. It has good diagnostic value. A score of less than 82 indicates likely dementia.

128 Correct Answer: B

Explanation: Signs and symptoms of carbon monoxide poisoning may include confusion, headache, dizziness, nausea or vomiting, shortness of breath and blurred vision. Carbon monoxide poisoning is caused by inhaling combustion fumes, which prevents oxygen from reaching your tissues and organs.

Reading

National Health Service. Carbon monoxide poisoning. www.nhs.uk/conditions/carbon-monoxide-poisoning/.

129 Correct Answer: C

Explanation: A direct question, such as asking the woman her father's age, can be confrontational to a person who struggles to find the correct answer. Reminding someone that a loved one has died may dig up feelings of grief, and challenging their perception of reality can be antagonistic. While steering someone onto a different topic can be helpful, negative answers like 'I can't. . .' may antagonise someone who feels trapped. When offering items to someone with advanced dementia, it may be better to give a choice of one or two items rather than a bigger range of options such as 'a drink'. Less complex sentences or questions are generally better. While challenging inaccurate information should be avoided, also reinforcing inaccuracies or telling lies is also unhelpful. In this situation, asking the woman about her father could be a chance to engage in some reminiscence.

Reading

The Alzheimer's Society website offers some advice on talking to people with dementia. www.alzheimers.org.uk/blog/language-dementia-what-not-to-say; www.alzheimers.org.uk/about-dementia/symptoms-and-diagnosis/symptoms/tips-for-communicating-dementia.

130 Correct Answer: A

Explanation: The question describes a dehydrated patient who is taking diuretics, with a low sodium of 115 mmol/L. The patient requires rehydration with an aim to correct the sodium deficit no faster than 12 mmol/24 hours, so the correct answer is intravenous sodium chloride solution 0.9%. There is no strong evidence for a urinary tract infection, and therefore oral antibiotics are not indicated. See NICE clinical knowledge summary 'Hyponatraemia' (2015).

131 Correct Answer: E

Explanation: Sodium valproate is used as an anticonvulsant and is also used in bipolar disorders as a mood stabiliser and in psychotic disorders, such as schizophrenia and schizoaffective disorder. Valproate encephalopathy is an important adverse side effect to recognise. It can be associated with normal liver function tests and normal serum sodium valproate levels. A raised ammonia level and recently starting this medication should raise suspicions for this diagnosis. As there is no alcohol history, no neurology and the liver function tests are normal, Wernicke's and hepatic encephalopathy are less likely. The urea and blood pressure are normal, making the other differentials less likely. Sodium valproate is considered safe with a wide therapeutic range. Potential adverse effects include dizziness, unsteadiness, headache, blurred vision and nystagmus, with tremor being the most common one affecting the central nervous system.

Reading

Farooq F, Sahib Din J, Khan AM, et al. Valproate-induced hyperammonemic encephalopathy. *Cureus* 2017; 9 (8).

NICE Clinical Knowledge Summary: Hyponatraemia, scenario: management (last revised in November 2020), https://cks.nice.org.uk/topics/hyponatraemia/management/management/

132 Correct Answer: B

Explanation: Structural neuroimaging in dementia can reveal atrophy decades prior to the onset of symptoms in cohorts of people with Mendelian forms of Alzheimer's disease and frontotemporal dementia. Nearly all the diagnostic criteria for neurodegenerative diseases now include neuroimaging as a supportive criterion, and in some cases, such as frontotemporal dementia, imaging changes are part of the core criteria. Different strengths of magnetic field are used according to need and provision. Currently, 1.5T scanners are most often used in clinical practice, and 3T MRI scanners are used for research at academic centres. The stronger magnetic field is particularly useful in identifying vascular abnormalities, including cerebral microbleeds, and obtaining better resolution of small structures in the brain, including subfields of the hippocampus.

Reading

Rittman T. Neurological update: Neuroimaging in dementia. *J Neurol* 2020; 267 (11): 3429–3435.

5

Continence

LEARNING OBJECTIVE:

To have the knowledge and skills required to assess and manage urinary and faecal incontinence and to articulate a continence service for a specific patient group in conjunction with nursing, therapy and surgical colleagues.

Areas to cover are:

- Anatomy and physiology of lower urinary tract and changes associated with later life.
- Pathophysiology of lower urinary tract and bowel disease in adults.
- Epidemiology, risk factors and causes of urinary and faecal incontinence.
- Treatment options for patients with bladder and bowel problems and the appropriate use of each.
- Rôle of the multidisciplinary team in the management of continence problems.
- Relevant recent research in continence in older people.
- Interpretation of the results of investigation in assessment, including frequency/volume chart, bladder scanning, urinalysis, multichannel cystometry or urodynamics, and anal ultrasound and manometry.
- Current evidence base and management options, including pharmacological treatments, behavioural treatments, surgical treatments, catheters and devices, padding and equipment.

- Application of the results of research to clinical practice.
- Design, implementation and development of integrated continence services.
- Rôle of continence nurse specialist, urogynacecologist and proctologist.

Questions

Question 133

An 83-year-old woman presents to the outpatient clinic with a complaint of urinary incontinence, which started three months ago. Which investigation is most likely to be helpful when assessing this woman for urinary incontinence?

A. 48-hour bladder diary

B. bladder scan

C. CT renal tract

D. cystoscopy

E. urinalysis

Question 134

A 73-year-old man is being assessed by the continence service. He reports dribbling small volumes of urine on multiple occasions during the day and overnight. His past history includes type 2 diabetes, for which he has been taking insulin for more than five years. A post-void bladder scan demonstrated a residual urine volume of over 400 mL. Cystometry and uroflowmetry tests are performed. Which of the following situations suggests bladder underactivity?

A. bladder pressure rise during a Valsalva manoeuvre

B. desire to pass urine after 300 mL have been instilled into the bladder

C. leakage of urine associated with detrusor contractions

D. maximum detrusor pressure 20 cm H_2O

E. maximum urine flow rate 50 mL per second

Question 135

An 80-year-old woman is seen in the continence service outpatient clinic along with her husband. She was diagnosed with Alzheimer's dementia over five years ago. She scored 12 out of 30 on a Montreal Cognitive Assessment test one month ago. They still live together in sheltered accommodation. Her husband reports that over the last few months she has developed episodes of faecal incontinence, and this causes both of them a great deal of distress. Regarding this woman's faecal incontinence, which of the following is most likely to be correct?

A. advice should be given about skin care and odour control

B. anorectal physiology studies should be performed

C. around one third of similar people also have urinary incontinence

D. pelvic muscle floor training is likely to be beneficial

E. stoma formation is a common first option in management

Question 136

A 90-year-old woman has severe Alzheimer's dementia and now resides in a nursing home. She has developed urinary incontinence, which was initially managed with pads, but she developed some excoriation of the perineal skin. This is causing her discomfort, and increased agitation has been noted by the care home staff. A urinary catheter was inserted but she pulled it out. Her current medication includes donepezil 10 mg daily. Physical examination does not reveal any other features. Her Montreal Cognitive Assessment score was 7 out of 30. Which of the following treatment strategies is most likely to be beneficial for this woman?

A. bladder anticholinergic medication

B. discontinue cholinesterase inhibitor

C. pelvic floor muscle training

D. prompted voiding strategy

E. reducing oral fluid intake

Question 137

Which of the following statements is most likely to be correct regarding ageing of the urinary tract?

A. a larger proportion of daily urine is formed at night

B. bladder M3 cholinergic receptor numbers increase

C. bladder wall collagen composition reduces

D. maximal detrusor contraction strength increases

E. renal urine concentrating ability is increased

Question 138

A 74-year-old woman has fallen several times overnight while trying to get to the toilet to pass urine. She reports nocturia on average three times per night. Her past medical history includes depression, hypertension and osteoporosis. She is taking numerous medications. On examination, she has a soft systolic heart murmur, there is mild bilateral ankle oedema and her chest and abdominal examinations are unremarkable. Her body mass index is calculated as 27 kg/m^2. Which of the following medications could be exacerbating her nocturia?

A. amlodipine

B. calcium and vitamin D supplement

C. indapamide

D. mirtazapine

E. ramipril

Question 139

A 78-year-old woman complains of having to get up four or five times each night to pass urine. On three occasions she has fallen overnight while trying to get out of bed. Which of the following lifestyle interventions is most likely to be beneficial for nocturia?

A. avoid caffeinated drinks in the hour before bedtime

B. elevate oedematous legs in the evenings

C. increase dietary salt intake

D. reduce total daily fluid intake

E. stop drinking alcohol in the hour before bedtime

Question 140

A 70-year-old woman complains of nocturia, having to get up to pass urine four or five times every night. She has been looking on the internet for something that might help and asks you about desmopressin. Which of the following statements regarding

desmopressin use for nocturia is most likely to be correct?

A. a reduction of two to three nocturia episodes per night is expected

B. an extension of sleep time before the first nocturia episode of around one hour is expected

C. daytime fluid intake should be increased while taking it

D. hypernatraemia occurs in 5% to 10% of people

E. it has to be administered as a nasal spray

Question 141

An 89-year-old woman is admitted following a fall. She has been taking 15 regular medications per day for a range of comorbidities. One of her medications is mirabegron, which has been prescribed for urge urinary incontinence episodes. Which of the following is true of mirabegron?

A. cognitive side effects are similar to anticholinergic drugs

B. discontinuation rates at 12 months are around 30% in real-life studies

C. orthostatic hypotension occurs in 5% to 10% of people

D. safety has been demonstrated in frail older people

E. the average reduction in incontinence episodes is smaller than with anticholinergic drugs

Question 142

A 93-year-old man lives alone in a ground floor flat. He normally mobilises independently with a four-wheeled walker the short distances around his property. His medical history includes hypertension, ischaemic heart disease and vascular Parkinsonism. Typically, he gets up three times a night to pass urine but also has had some episodes of urinary incontinence. He has fallen on several occasions while getting out of bed or getting on and off the toilet. Which continence aid would be most useful to try for this man?

A. bed pan

B. bedside commode

C. in-dwelling urinary catheter

D. raised toilet seat and armrest surround

E. urine bottle

Question 143

You assess an older man in the outpatient clinic who complains of problems passing water. Regarding lower urinary tract symptoms in men, which of the following would best indicate a problem with urine storage?

A. incomplete bladder emptying

B. nocturia

C. poor urine flow

D. post-micturition dribbling

E. start hesitancy

Question 144

A 79-year-old woman reports episodes of incontinence. While awaiting further assessment and a longer-term management plan, she is keen to try some form of containment aid and asks for your advice. Which of the following statements is correct regarding continence containment pads?

A. all products have a standardised absorbency rating scale

B. barrier creams help protect the skin from faecal incontinence

C. disposable pads are more cost effective than washable ones

D. modern washable pads have a super-absorbent polymer powder core

E. pull-up style pants are elasticated so that one size fits all

Question 145

A 65-year-old woman with a history of multiple sclerosis has been admitted to the rehabilitation unit. She has developed urinary incontinence and finds this embarrassing. She has heard of a treatment where a drug is injected into the bladder and asks if it is an option for her. Which of the following is true regarding the use of botulinum toxin type A for the treatment of urinary incontinence?

A. a maximal symptom benefit occurs within one week of injections

B. injections need to be repeated every two to three months

C. it is a first-line treatment option for neurogenic detrusor overactivity

D. prophylactic antibiotics negate the risk of procedure-related urinary tract infection

E. the average reduction in urinary incontinence episodes is similar to that achieved with oral anticholinergic medications

Question 146

An 83-year-old woman attends a falls clinic. She gives a history suggestive of urge urinary incontinence and has a normal post voiding bladder scan. Her daughter states that whenever she gets one of 'her UTIs' she is confused and sleepy. Concerned by her potential for delirium, you are cautious regarding her medication. Which of the following carries the lowest anticholinergic burden?

A. mirabegron

B. oxybutynin

C. solifenacin

D. tolterodine

E. trospium

Question 147

A 65-year-old woman presents to the clinic with symptoms of urge incontinence. She has tried limiting her consumption of caffeine and soft drinks, especially in the evenings, although this has not made a significant difference to her symptoms. She has no past medical history of note and takes no regular medication. There are no significant findings on physical examination. Her body mass index is 22 kg/m². Which of the following is the most appropriate next step?

A. bladder training

B. duloxetine

C. finasteride

D. mirabegron

D. oxybutynin

Answers for Chapter 5

133 Correct Answer: B

Explanation: Bladder diaries should be for a minimum of 72 hours. A bladder scan to assess for residual urine volume is helpful but other imaging of the renal tract is not usually required, and neither is cystoscopy. Urinalysis to look for evidence of urinary tract infection is not recommended in people aged over 65.

Reading

National Institute for Health and Care Excellence. Urinary incontinence and pelvic organ prolapse in women: Management (NG123). 2019. www.nice.org.uk/guidance/ng123.

134 Correct Answer: D

Explanation: Post-void residual volume can be measured by ultrasound scanning. A postvoid residual of 100 millilitres or more can be a sign that the bladder is not emptying completely, but in older people a value up to 200 mL may be acceptable. Cystometry is performed with a specialised catheter inserted into the bladder, which can be used to slowly instil water and can also measure pressure change. A pressure sensor can also be inserted into the rectum to measure intra-abdominal pressure concurrently. Subtracting abdominal pressure readings from bladder readings can evaluate detrusor contractions. Uroflowmetry measures urine flow rate and the volume passed. It requires urinating into a specialised measuring funnel. This produces a graph showing flow rate over time. A low flow rate suggests impaired bladder contraction or outflow obstruction. It can be performed following cystometry with the pressure sensors still in place to evaluate detrusor activity along with urine flow. A bladder pressure rise during a Valsalva manoeuvre is normal (subtract from intra-abdominal pressure). A strong desire to pass urine after 300 mL have been instilled is expected. Detrusor contractions causing urine leakage suggest overactivity. A maximal detrusor pressure of 20 cm H_2O suggests underactivity. A maximal flow rate of 50 mL per second is not impaired.

135 Correct Answer: A

Explanation: Around two thirds of people with faecal incontinence also have urinary incontinence, termed 'dual incontinence'. Better management may improve quality of life and delay the need for 24-hour care placement, but this might ultimately be required. Risk factors relevant to older people include frailty, cognitive impairment, neurological disorders (e.g. stroke), urinary incontinence and pelvic organ prolapse. Management strategies may target reduced mobility, faecal loading and diarrhoea. Cauda equina syndrome is a possibility. Loperamide is used first line for diarrhoea control; codeine phosphate is a second line option. Body-worn pads, possibly also bed pads, should be provided. Anal plugs are an option, if tolerated. Advice should be given on skin care and odour control. Specialist continence services might offer pelvic floor muscle training, bowel retraining, specialist dietary assessment and management, biofeedback, electrical stimulation and rectal irrigation. Cognitive impairment is likely to limit how the woman in the scenario benefits. Further testing and surgical interventions are occasionally beneficial for selected people. Specialist investigations can include anorectal physiology studies, endoanal/endovaginal/perineal ultrasound and proctography. Surgical options include sphincter repair, temporary sacral nerve stimulation, neosphincter (i.e. stimulated graciloplasty or an artificial anal sphincter) and stoma formation (the last resort).

Reading

National Institute for Health and Care Excellence. Faecal incontinence in adults: Management. Clinical Guideline 49, 2007. www.nice.org.uk/guidance/cg49.

136 Correct Answer: B

Explanation: Bladder anticholinergic medications may worsen her cognition. Also, only oxybutynin has been tested in a nursing home population, and it was ineffective for urinary incontinence. Cholinesterase inhibitors can cause urinary incontinence. Given her advanced dementia and nursing home residence, the benefits of continuing this drug are limited. Discontinuation should be tried given her current distress. She is unlikely to be able to effectively perform pelvic floor exercises. Prompted voiding has limited evidence of benefit. Reducing fluid intake will not help; in fact, limited evidence suggests increasing fluid intake might be helpful.

Reading

Starr JM. Cholinesterase inhibitor treatment and urinary incontinence in Alzheimer's disease. *J Am Geriatr Soc* 2007; 55: 800–801.

Wagg A, Gibson W, Ostaszkiewicz J, et al. Urinary incontinence in frail elderly persons: Report from the 5th International Consultation on Incontinence. *Neurourol Urodyn* 2015; 34: 398–406.

137 Correct Answer: A

Explanation: Bladder wall collagen composition increases and muscle composition declines in older age. The result is a stiffer bladder that is more difficult to fully empty. M3 cholinergic receptor numbers are reduced. Renal urine concentrating ability declines, increasing the risk of dehydration. Diurnal variation in urine production becomes blunted, leading to more urine being produced at night.

Reading

Gibson W, Wagg A. New horizons: Urinary incontinence in older people. *Age Ageing* 2014; 43: 157–163.

138 Correct Answer: A

Explanation: Calcium channel blockers (CCB) have been associated with the development of nocturia. It has been speculated that reabsorption of peripheral oedema, caused as a side effect of CCB treatment, overnight could increase intravascular volume and precipitate the urge to go. However, some people without peripheral oedema can also develop nocturia. A withdrawal of amlodipine should be considered for this woman.

Reading

Santiapillai J, Tadtayev S, Miles A, et al. Dihydropyridine calcium channel blockers and obstructive sleep apnea: Two underrecognized causes of nocturia? *Neurourol Urodyn* 2020; 39: 1612–1614.

139 Correct Answer: B

Explanation: 'Clinically significant' nocturia is often defined as two or more episodes of urination interrupting sleep. With older age comes loss of the diurnal variation in vasopressin secretion, leading to a greater proportion of urine being formed at night. A reduced bladder capacity may also contribute. Comorbidities such as obstructive sleep apnoea, heart failure and polyuria (e.g. due to diabetes) may play a rôle in some people. It is an important potential contributor to nocturnal falls. Relevant lifestyle advice includes avoid alcohol and caffeine, do not drink any fluids in the two hours before bed, elevate legs in evenings if they are oedematous and restrict dietary salt.

Reading

Monaghan TF, Michelson KP, Wu ZD, et al. Sodium restriction improves nocturia in patients at a cardiology clinic. *J Clin Hypertens* 2020; 22: 633–638.

140 Correct Answer: B

Explanation: Desmopressin is a synthetic analogue of vasopressin, which has an antidiuretic effect. It is available in oral tablet, sublingual and intranasal formulations. Trial data suggest approximately 0.5 fewer voids per night and one hour longer sleep duration before first void compared to placebo. Hyponatraemia is a recognised side effect (relative risk 5.1, 95% CI 3.0 to 8.8) with an incidence highest after around two to three weeks of therapy. Desmopressin should be discontinued if serum sodium drops below the normal range. Users need to fluid restrict concurrently and avoid other medications that could induce SIADH (e.g. antidepressants and carbamazepine). Given the risk of side effects, it is unlikely to be suitable for frail older people with nocturia.

Reading

Desmopressin for nocturia in adults. *Drug Ther Bull* March 2017; 55 (3). doi: 10.1136/dtb.2017.3.0460.

141 Correct Answer: E

Explanation: Mirabegron is a beta-3 adrenoceptor agonist that promotes bladder relaxation. It should not cause cognitive side effects but does have a small increased risk of hypertension and tachycardia. However, the drug has not been tested in frail older people. Around 70% to 90% of people discontinue mirabegron within the first 12 months of prescription (a figure similar to anticholinergic drugs). The average reduction in daily urinary incontinence episodes is around 0.4, compared to 0.6 for bladder anticholinergics.

Reading

Cui Y, Zong H, Yang C, et al. The efficacy and safety of mirabegron in treating OAB: A systematic review and meta-analysis of phase III trials. *Int Urol Nephrol* 2014; 46: 275–284.

Samuelsson E, Odeberg J, Stenzelius K, et al. Effect of pharmacological treatment for urinary incontinence in the elderly and frail elderly: A systematic review. *Geriatr Gerontol Int* 2015; 15: 521–534.

Kinjo M, Sekiguchi Y, Yoshimura Y, et al. Long-term persistence with mirabegron versus solifenacin in women with overactive bladder: Prospective, randomized trial. *LUTS* 2018; 10: 148–152.

142 Correct Answer: E

Explanation:

Bed pan—useful if person cannot get out of bed. Needs to be placed beneath them, which can require more than one person to assist. The unnatural position makes bowel motions difficult. A slipper pan, with a sloped side, can be easier to place under people with reduced ability to raise their hips off the bed.

Commode—useful if person has difficulty mobilising the distance to the toilet, e.g. placed at bedside for overnight use.

Urine bottle—typically for less mobile men to use when in bed, requires some dexterity and cognitive ability. Female versions designed mainly for wheelchair users are available.

Raised toilet seat—easier to get on and off the toilet but reduces the natural squatting position for defaecation.

Toilet surround—sits around the toilet and provides armrests of adjustable height to help getting on and off the toilet.

Catheter—this would increase his risk of urinary tract infections and may reduce his mobilisation; it should not be the first thing to try.

143 Correct Answer: B

Explanation: Voiding symptoms—e.g. start hesitancy, weak/intermittent flow of urine, the need to strain, terminal dribbling and incomplete emptying.

• *Storage symptoms*—e.g. urgency, frequency, nocturia and incontinence.

• *Post-micturition symptoms*—e.g. dribbling.

Thought to affect around 30% of men aged over 65 years.

Symptom severity can be quantified by the International Prostate Symptom Score: 0–7 'mild', 8–19 'moderate' and 20–35 rated 'severe'.

Reading

National Institute for Health and Care Excellence. Lower urinary tract symptoms in men: Management. Clinical Guideline 97, 2010. www.nice.org.uk/guidance/cg97.

144 Correct Answer: B

Explanation: Washable pads are usually more cost effective than disposable ones if they can be reused multiple times (probably not for faecal incontinence); they do not contribute as much to landfill but do require laundry. Absorbency can be hard to establish without trying different pads (the 'Rothwell method' tests fluid absorbency volume in laboratory conditions but isn't an industry standard). Bigger pads tend to absorb more fluid but are less discrete. Mobile and independent people may prefer smaller pads that they change frequently, especially in social situations. Disposable pads have a top sheet to keep the skin dry, an absorbent core (i.e. fluffed wood pulp fibres mixed with a super-absorbent polymer powder) and a waterproof backing. Washable pads can be traditional terry towelling (cotton) or more modern forms with three layers similar to the disposable ones. The absorbent core is made of a washable material such as felt. Fitted pads (e.g. pull-up style pants) come in a range of sizes as well as absorbency ratings. Pant-liner style pads with an adhesive backing are a more discrete option. Thinner pads might be ok for people who have bowel leakage alone, as less fluid often needs to be absorbed. With faecal incontinence, a barrier cream might help to protect the skin (but change pad ASAP), and washable pads are usually not appropriate.

Reading

Continence Product Advisor. www.continenceproductadvisor.org/products.

145 Correct Answer: E

Explanation: Botulinum toxin type A can be injected into the bladder wall using a cystoscope. The procedure takes around 30 minutes and is usually done as an outpatient under local anaesthetic. Twenty to 30 sites are injected around the bladder (typically sparing the trigone). Symptom improvement is not expected until two weeks after the procedure and it needs to be repeated every 6 to 12 months. It is associated with an increased risk of UTI. Prophylactic antibiotics for a few days either side of the procedure can reduce but do not remove this risk. Urinary retention is another potential complication. It is usually considered when other treatment options have failed. Data suggest a similar effect size in reducing daily episodes of urinary incontinence compared to oral anticholinergic drugs.

Reading

Karsenty G, Baverstock R, Carlson K, et al. Technical aspects of botulinum toxin type A injection in the bladder to treat urinary incontinence: Reviewing the procedure. *Int J Clin Pract* 2014; 68: 731–742.

Visco AG, Zyczynski H, Brubaker L, et al. Cost-effectiveness analysis of anticholinergics vs. Botox for urgency urinary incontinence: Results from the ABC randomized trial. *Female Pelvic Med Reconstr Surg* 2016; 22: 311–316.

146 Correct Answer: A

Explanation: Mirabegron is a β_3-adrenoreceptor agonist that represents an alternative treatment to antimuscarinics in terms of anticholinergic burden.

Reading

Griebling TL, Campbell NL, Mangel J, et al. Effect of mirabegron on cognitive function in elderly patients with overactive bladder: MoCA results from a phase 4 randomized, placebo-controlled study (PILLAR). *BMC Geriatr* 2020; 20 (1): 109.

147 Correct Answer: A

Explanation: Bladder training, with a planned gradual increase in the interval between trips to the toilet for voiding, is the most appropriate next step. Women with symptoms of urgency or mixed urinary incontinence are offered bladder training for a minimum of six weeks as first-line treatment. Bladder training teaches a woman how to hold more urine in her bladder and so reduce the number of times she needs to pass urine. It also includes lifestyle advice on the amount and types of fluids to drink and coping strategies to reduce urgency.

Reading

Urinary incontinence in women. Quality standard [QS77]. January 2015. www.nice.org.uk/guidance/qs77/chapter/Quality-statement-5-Bladder-training.

6

Falls and Poor Mobility

Falls

LEARNING OBJECTIVE:

To know how to assess and manage older patients presenting with falls (with or without fracture) and syncope in an acute or community setting.

Areas to cover are:

- Appreciation that causes of falls are often multifactorial.
- Models of falls prevention services, including referral to appropriate services, e.g. exercise classes, tilt testing.
- Health promotion.
- Ability to diagnose causes and risk factors for falls.
- Risk factors, consequences and impact of falls.
- Drug and neurovascular causes of falls and syncope.
- Assessment of falls (including causes such as syncope, postural hypotension, cardiac arrhythmias, carotid sinus syndrome, vertigo including BPPV, dizziness, poor vision, drugs/polypharmacy).
- Medication review.
- Assessment of gait, balance and vision, including using at least one validated balance assessment tool.
- Epidemiology of syncope.
- Aetiology and pathophysiology of syncope.

- Evidence-based assessment and treatment of syncope (including ECG, cardiac monitors, event recorders/Holter, echocardiogram, BP evaluation, tilt testing and carotid sinus massage).
- Assessment or diagnosis of and treatment of dizziness and vertigo (including Dix-Hallpike test and Epley manoeuvre, and consent for procedures).
- Assessment of bone health (including interpretation of bone density scans and use at least one validated tool) and treatment of osteoporosis and vitamin D deficiency.
- Assessment of functional ability and need for rehabilitation.
- Evidence-based interventions to prevent falls or reduce falls risk and to minimise consequences, e.g. use of care alarms.
- Multidisciplinary approach (e.g. PT, OT, risk assessment, environment).
- Awareness of compromises between patient's safety and improved mobility.
- The importance of the 'fear of falling syndrome'.

- Relevant national and international publications, guidelines and audits, e.g. NICE, AGS/BGS/AAOS, Cochrane review, national audit.

Poor mobility

LEARNING OBJECTIVE:

To know how to assess the cause of immobility and declining mobility and aid its management.

Areas to cover are:

- Risk factors and causes of immobility.
- Assessment including physical examination (including risk factors and causes) of declining mobility or immobility (including osteoarthrosis, inflammatory arthritis, crystal arthropathies, polymyalgia rheumatica, myositis and myopathy, cervical and lumbar myelopathy).
- Assessment of patients presenting with immobility or declining mobility (including risk factors and causes).
- Gait assessment.
- Drug and non-drug interventions to improve mobility and prevent immobility.

Questions

Question 148

An 86-year-old widow presented as an outpatient, with her son. She had experienced three falls in the previous year, none with any associated palpations or chest pain. She had a past history of osteoarthritis which limited her mobility, hypertension, ischaemic heart disease, urinary incontinence and anxiety. She lived alone and was afraid to go out very much. She was taking aspirin, ramipril, bendroflumethiazide, verapamil, escitalopram and oxybutynin. She was also taking pseudoephedrine as a cough medicine which she had bought over the counter. What is the next most appropriate step in the assessment of her falls?

A. gait and balance assessment

B. 24-hour electrocardiogram monitoring

C. medication review

D. serum electrolyte measurement

E. tilt-table test

Question 149

A 70-year-old woman presents to the falls clinic, complaining of a sudden and transient loss of consciousness, which subsided spontaneously and without a localising neurological deficit. She had been to the GP recently with a three-month history of 'dizziness'. She described several episodes of the room spinning around her. These typically lasted between two hours and a whole day. She felt tired after these attacks. She has noticed progressive hearing loss. No diagnosis had been made. She had a past history of glaucoma and hypertension. What is the next most appropriate step to help with diagnosis?

A. audiology review
B. ENT review
C. Epley manoeuvre
D. restriction of salt, caffeine or alcohol intake
E. vestibular rehabilitation

Question 150

Which of the following statements concerning muscle and sarcopenia is true?

A. IL-10, an anti-inflammatory cytokine, declines in the human circulation with age
B. it is generally accepted that low physical performance is defined as any gait speed of less than 1.6 m/sec
C. the function of 'satellite cells' in sarcopenia is normal
D. the relationship between loss of muscle mass and loss of muscle strength is best described as linear
E. there is little evidence from human studies of sarcopenia to suggest that loss of muscle mass is primarily driven by a blunted synthetic response to both feeding and exercise

Question 151

Which of the following states concerning postural or orthostatic hypotension is true?

A. antigravity suits are commonly useful in management
B. cardiac pacemakers are a first-line treatment for postural hypotension due to chronic neurogenic failure
C. drugs are needed when non-pharmacological approaches are unsuccessful
D. postural (orthostatic) hypotension is defined as a fall in blood pressure of over 10 mmHg systolic (or 5 mmHg diastolic), on standing or during head-up tilt to at least 60°
E. the generalised use of home blood pressure monitoring should be encouraged

Question 152

Prolonged standing, change in posture and hot environments are common precipitating factors for vasovagal syncope (VVS). Which of the following statements about VVS is also true?

A. older people are significantly more likely to report prolonged standing, change in posture and hot environments as precipitating factors for VVS compared to younger people
B. patients should be advised to ensure adequate hydration and to avoid possible precipitants
C. the classic prodrome always accompanies VVS
D. there is no reliable diagnostic test to support a diagnosis of VVS
E. VVS is relatively uncommon as a diagnosis in older people

Question 153

In a falls clinic, an 84-year-old female complains, 'Doctor, I feel funny whenever I turn in bed at night, or I hang the washing on the line'. She later reports that these episodes have occurred in bouts lasting several weeks and will then spontaneously remit, only to return weeks, months or even years later. A diagnosis, using the Dix-Hallpike manoeuvre, of benign paroxysmal positional vertigo (BPPV) is made. What is the most common cause of BPPV?

A. head trauma
B. idiopathic
C. inner ear surgery

D. Ménière's disease

E. viral labyrinthitis

Question 154

Fear of falling (FOF) has been identified as one of the key components of the 'falls syndrome'. Which of the following statements is true regarding FOF?

A. FOF is not a suitable target for intervention in falls prevention programmes

B. FOF is only found in patients who have experienced a fall

C. it is straightforward to develop an instrument that fully reflects a broad view of FOF

D. the Falls Efficacy Scale assesses the degree of perceived self-efficacy at avoiding a fall during basic activities of daily living

E. there is no effect of age on FOF

Question 155

Drugs commonly known to cause postural hypotension include:

A. ACE inhibitors

B. anticonvulsants

C. benzodiazepines

D. codeine-based analgesics

E. opiates

Question 156

An 82-year-old retired teacher, with no other symptoms, consults to the falls clinic with a history of frequent stumbling and numbness of the upper side of her left foot. She reports confinement to bed, but otherwise she has had no other symptoms. A diagnosis of left foot drop is made. What is the most likely cause?

A. cauda equina syndrome

B. L5 radiculopathy

C. peroneal neuropathy

D. polio

E. stroke

Question 157

Which of the following symptoms makes syncope more likely than a seizure?

A. automatisms such as chewing or lip smacking

B. blueness of the face

C. hemi-lateral clonic movements

D. light-headedness or blurring of vision

E. tongue biting

Question 158

Regarding people identified as being at increased risk of falling following a multifactorial assessment, which of the following is recommended as part of successful intervention strategies?

A. brisk walking

B. hip protectors

C. home hazard assessment and intervention

D. referral for correction of visual impairment as a single intervention

E. vitamin D supplementation

Question 159

Regarding podiatry interventions to prevent falls in older people, which one of the following statements is true?

A. lack of participant and intervention provider blinding can be a source of bias

B. podiatry interventions have no effect on falls of older people living in their own homes

C. referral to podiatry services has no effect on falls frequency

D. the likelihood of falls for people living in care homes is about the same as the likelihood of falls for older people living in the community

E. there is little need for trials of podiatry interventions to reduce falls in care homes

Question 160

Which one of the following changes is thought to occur in ageing muscle?

A. increase in size of motor units

B. increased mitochondrial activity

C. increased muscle protein synthesis

D. increased oxidative stress

E. reduction in non-contractile proteins

Question 161

An 86-year-old female patient has had a number of falls and is referred to the falls clinic. After some initial consideration, she is considered for a trans-catheter aortic valve implantation (TAVI). She has had a confirmed diagnosis of severe, symptomatic aortic stenosis, and her case has been discussed at the TAVI multidisciplinary team (MDT). She is considered extreme risk for surgical aortic valve replacement (owing to her age, frailty and comorbidities), but the TAVI may be beneficial due to the patient's medical characteristics and circumstances. Which of the following statements is true?

A. a number of surgical risk scores have been validated to assess risk for TAVI insertion in the older population

B. severe pulmonary hypertension might incline an MDT towards intervention

C. the potential improvement in quality of life following TAVI, as determined by the MDT, in light of the comorbidities would not be a consideration for a TAVI

D. the presence of an extensive aortic calcification ('porcelain aorta') might incline towards surgery instead

E. trans-thoracic echocardiography is considered an essential part of the work-up for a TAVI

Question 162

A 71-year-old man experiences another transient loss of consciousness, witnessed by some onlookers also in the pub. He and the witnesses were asked to describe what happened before, during and after the event, an ECG was recorded, and a full history and examination were subsequently completed. In which one of the following might a referral to assess the possibility of psychogenic non-epileptic seizures rather than a cardiovascular assessment be warranted?

A. evidence of a short QT syndrome

B. heart failure (history or physical signs)

C. multiple unexplained physical symptoms

D. new or unexplained breathlessness

E. transient loss of consciousness during exertion

Question 163

An 82-year-old female, with no known significant other medical conditions apart from mild untreated hypertension, presents to the falls clinic, having 'tripped on a rug'. She reports dizziness, nausea and light-headedness about two hours after meals. Following investigations, a tentative diagnosis of post-prandial hypotension (PPH) is made. Which of the following statements is true about PPH?

A. in most cases there is a dominant aetiological factor in PPH

B. it is a consistent finding that withholding antihypertensive therapy improves the falls frequency in patients experiencing PPH

C. of the macronutrients, glucose appears to elicit the least rapid decrease in systolic BP in healthy older subjects

D. PPH has been rigorously studied well

E. PPH has been traditionally defined as a fall in systolic BP of >20 mmHg, or a decrease to <90 mmHg when the pre-prandial BP is <100 mmHg, within two hours of a meal

Question 164

Which of the following statements is true concerning balance and gait impairment screening tests in the older patient visiting primary care?

A. an ability to turn without staggering is of note in the 'Timed Up and Go' test

B. higher scores on the Tinetti Falls Efficacy Scale indicate greater confidence in walking

C. in the 'Timed Up and Go' test, the patient is asked to walk barefoot without any mobility aids

D. the normal time required to complete the 'Timed Up and Go' test is anything below 20 seconds

E. the Tinetti Fall Efficacy Scale is a 20-item questionnaire

Question 165

A 92-year-old presents to falls clinic with a few episodes of syncope. He only complains of 'tripping over a mobile rug'. On deeper questioning, he complains of a few months' history of severe, paroxysmal episodes of pain, localised to the left external ear canal and the base of the tongue. The pain is sharp, stabbing

and severe and is associated with intervening periods of a low-grade dull ache. It is even precipitated by coughing. He does not report any syncopal episodes triggered by lateral neck movement or shaving. Examination including full neurological examination in clinic was normal. No 'trigger zone' is found.

What is the most likely underlying diagnosis?

A. carotid sinus hypersensitivity

B. cough syncope

C. micturition syncope

D. trigeminal neuralgia

E. vasoglossopharyngeal neuralgia

Question 166

What is the level of unintentional weight loss compared to last year, in kilograms, considered 'abnormal', according to the Fried criteria for frailty, obtained from the patient, carer or medical records?

A. >1

B. >3

C. >5

D. >10

E. >15

Question 167

A 69-year-old woman taking atorvastatin for the past nine months after a coronary bypass grafting presents with progressive, symmetrical, proximal muscle weakness and pain. She describes symptoms in both legs and to a lesser extent in both arms starting in the week prior to presentation. Biochemical analysis showed a markedly elevated creatine kinase (24,159 U/L). The statin was discontinued and therapy for rhabdomyolysis was commenced in the intensive care unit.

What is the most likely diagnosis?

TABLE 6.1

Investigations.

Serology	Epstein-Barr, herpes simplex, cytomegalo- and adenovirus, hepatitis B and C virus, HIV, mycoplasma, Coxsackie, (para)influenza, and Echinococcus showed no significant abnormalities
Tumour markers	CA 125 and CA 19.9 normal
Anti-Jo-1 antibodies	Negative
Anti-HMGCR antibodies	Highly elevated
Muscle biopsy	Mild inflammatory changes and marked necrotic muscle fibre

A. anti-synthetase syndrome

B. dermatomyositis

C. immune-mediated necrotising myopathy

D. inclusion body myositis

E. viral myositis

Question 168

A 78-year-old man is admitted to hospital after being found on his bedroom floor. He has a background of presumed Alzheimer's disease and cannot recall the events. He has presented to hospital four times in the last year due to falls. On examination, there is minor bruising to both knees. His current medications include alendronate 70 mg weekly and diazepam 2 mg tds. Which of the following assessments is *least* useful?

A. assessment of cognitive impairment

B. assessment of continence

C. detailed falls history

D. inpatient falls risk prediction tool

E. medication review

Question 169

An 80-year-old man reports deteriorating mobility over the last six months. Both knees are painful when he walks and this limits his mobility. Physical examination reveals Heberden's nodes, and there is significant crepitus present at both knee joints. His BMI is calculated as 42 kg/m². Which of the following measures would be most appropriate?

A. acupuncture

B. chondroitin supplements

C. glucosamine supplements

D. regular oral ibuprofen

E. regular oral paracetamol

Question 170

An 82-year-old woman presented after a sudden blackout. She had been standing in a queue at the post office for five minutes when she started to feel dizzy and unwell. She felt sweaty and clammy and had then lost consciousness. A witness described her falling to the floor, after which she appeared very pale and intermittently jerked her arms. She was unconscious for approximately three minutes. When she regained consciousness, she was orientated quickly and able to talk normally with the witness. She had a history of hypertension, for which she was taking amlodipine 5 mg daily and ramipril 5 mg daily. On examination, her pulse was 72 beats/min and regular, and her BP was 135/60 mmHg supine and 120/60 mmHg after standing for three minutes. She had normal heart sounds, and neurological examination was normal.

What is the most appropriate next step in management?

TABLE 6.2

Investigations.

Haemoglobin	146 g/L (115–165)
Serum sodium	143 mmol/L (137–144)
Serum potassium	4.4 mmol/L (3.5–5.0)
ECG	PR interval 124 ms (120–200), QTc interval 420 ms (300–450), QRS duration 119 ms

A. ambulatory ECG recording

B. echocardiography

C. MRI scan of brain

D. no further investigation

E. tilt-table test

Question 171

A 70-year-old man who is independently mobile and lives with his son presents with a sudden fall accompanied by a burning back pain. Past history includes diet-controlled diabetes, hypertension and atrial fibrillation. In the previous days, he had been suffering from a lower respiratory tract infection for which his GP had commenced a five-day course of amoxicillin. The patient was on the last day of his treatment and was recovering from his symptoms when his legs gave way beneath him as he stood up. He was unable to get up thereafter and his son called for an ambulance. On examination, his lower limbs are areflexic with bilateral extensor plantars. A sensory level is detected at the umbilicus. Proprioception and vibration sense are intact. Power is 2/5 in the lower limbs and 5/5 in the upper limbs. Which of the following is the most likely diagnosis in this case?

A. cauda equina syndrome

B. side effect of amoxicillin

C. spinal cord compression

D. spinal cord infarction

E. transverse myelitis

Answers for Chapter 6

148 Correct Answer: C

Explanation: The patient is taking more than five medications; this constitutes polypharmacy, which can be a common cause of falls in older people. A recent study has shown that almost one third of the total population uses five or more drugs, which was significantly associated with 21% increased rate of falls over a two-year period. Gait and balance assessment may be indicated at some stage in the assessment, but the episodes are infrequent so it may not be helpful. The patient does not have a history of syncope, palpations or chest pain, reducing the justification for a 24-hour ECG.

Reading

Dhalwani NN, Fahami R, Sathanapally H, et al. Association between polypharmacy and falls in older adults: A longitudinal study from England. *BMJ Open* 2017; 7: e016358.

149 Correct Answer: B

Explanation: The concern is that the patient has Ménière's disease evidenced by recurrent episodes of vertigo, associated with hearing loss. There is no evidence from randomised controlled trials to support or refute the restriction of salt, caffeine or alcohol intake in patients with Ménière's disease. The Epley manoeuvre would be useful in treating benign paroxysmal positional vertigo but not Ménière's disease. The diagnosis needs to be confirmed before vestibular rehabilitation.

Reading

Hussain K, Murdin L, Schilder AG. Restriction of salt, caffeine and alcohol intake for the treatment of Ménière's disease or syndrome. *Cochrane Database Syst Rev* 2018; 12 (12): CD012173.

Pyykkö I, Manchaiah V, Zou J, Levo H, Kentala E. Do patients with Ménière's disease have attacks of syncope? *J Neurol* 2017; 264 (Suppl 1): 48–54.

150 Correct Answer: A

Explanation: IL-10, an anti-inflammatory cytokine, declines in the circulation with age in humans. But the other statements are incorrect. Although somewhat arbitrary, it is generally accepted that low physical performance is defined as a gait speed of less than 0.8 m/sec. Whilst loss of muscle mass is associated with loss of muscle strength, the relationship is not linear. The majority of studies investigating sarcopenia in humans have suggested that loss of muscle mass is primarily driven by a blunted synthetic response to both feeding and exercise, termed 'anabolic resistance'. Sarcopenia is developed by unbalanced protein synthesis and degradation as well as dysfunction of satellite cells.

Reading

Park SS, Kwon ES, Kwon KS. Molecular mechanisms and therapeutic interventions in Sarcopenia. *Osteoporos Sarcopenia* 2017; 3 (3): 117–122.

Wilson D, Jackson T, Sapey E, et al. Frailty and sarcopenia: The potential role of an aged immune system. *Ageing Res Rev* 2017; 36: 1–10.

151 Correct Answer: C

Explanation: Drugs are needed when non-pharmacological approaches are unsuccessful. The generalised use of home blood pressure monitoring should be discouraged because of the variability of blood pressure, its propensity to change rapidly and difficulties with accurate recording, especially when low. Postural (orthostatic) hypotension is defined as a fall in blood pressure of over 20 mmHg systolic (or 10 mmHg diastolic), on standing or during head-up tilt to at least 60°. Small, frequent meals ensure an adequate caloric intake and reduce postprandial hypotension. Antigravity suits have virtually no rôle. Cardiac pacemakers have no place in postural hypotension due to chronic neurogenic failure.

Reading

Mathias CJ, Kimber JR. Treatment of postural hypotension. *J Neurol Neurosurg Psychiatry* 1998; 65 (3): 285–289.

152 Correct Answer: B

Explanation: VVS is a common diagnosis in older people. Patients could be advised to ensure adequate hydration and to avoid possible precipitants. VVS in the older patient was assumed rare until head-up tilt-table testing was described by Kenny et al. (1986) as a diagnostic tool for VVS. The classical prodrome of pallor, sweatiness, nausea, abdominal discomfort, dizziness or light-headedness often accompanies VVS. In the older patient, however, this prodrome is more likely to be short or even non-existent. In one study, however, older patients have been significantly less likely to report the above symptoms (Duncan et al., 2010).

Reading

Duncan GW, Tan MP, Newton JL, et al. Vasovagal syncope in the older person: Differences in presentation between older and younger patients. *Age Ageing* 2010; 39 (4): 465–470.

Kenny RA, Ingram A, Bayliss J, et al. Head-up tilt:
    A useful test for investigating unexplained syncope.
    Lancet 1986; 1 (8494): 1352–1355.
Tan MP, Parry SW. Vasovagal syncope in the older
    patient. *J Am Coll Cardiol* 2008; 51 (6): 599–606.

153 Correct Answer: B

Explanation: Epidemiology varies, but one source (Parnes et al., 2003) cites causes of BPPV as primary or idiopathic (50%–70%) or secondary (30%–50%) (causes including head trauma (7%–17%), viral labyrinthitis (15%), Ménière's disease (5%), migraines (<5%), and inner ear surgery [<1%]). Different studies vary, but idiopathic causes comprise the largest group of patients.

Reading

Halmagyi GM, Cremer PD. Assessment and treatment
    of dizziness. *J Neurol Neurosurg Psychiatry* 2000;
    68 (2): 129–134.
Parnes LS, Agrawal SK, Atlas J. Diagnosis and man-
    agement of benign paroxysmal positional vertigo
    (BPPV). *CMAJ* 2003; 169 (7): 681–693.

154 Correct Answer: D

Explanation: The Falls Efficacy Scale assesses the degree of perceived self-efficacy at avoiding a fall during basic activities of daily living. Prevalence of FOF appears to increase with age and to be higher in women. Because of the many differently measured risk factors that contribute to FOF and the consequences of FOF, it may be difficult to develop an instrument that fully reflects a broad view of FOF. FOF is also commonly found among older people who have not yet experienced a fall. FOF is one of the potential modifiable risk factors where interventions could be effective in the prevention of falls.

Reading

Scheffer AC, Schuurmans MJ, van Dijk N, et al. Fear
    of falling: Measurement strategy, prevalence, risk
    factors and consequences among older persons. *Age
    Ageing* 2008; 37 (1): 19–24.

155 Correct Answer: A

Explanation: Drugs linked to falls causation are listed in Table 6.3.

Reading

Anderson KE. Falls in the elderly. *J R Coll Physicians
    Edinb* 2008; 38: 138–143.

156 Correct Answer: C

Explanation: The most common cause of spontaneous foot drop is peroneal neuropathy, often as a result of compression at the neck of the fibula at knee level, where the common peroneal nerve is

TABLE 6.3

Drugs linked to falls.

Drugs linked to falls by causing postural hypotension	Drugs linked to falls via other mechanisms, e.g. sedation/confusion/unsteadiness
Nitrates	Benzodiazepines
ACE inhibitors	Antipsychotics
Anticholinergics	Opiates
L-dopa	Codeine-based analgesics
Antiplatelet agents	Anticonvulsants
Antidepressants, particularly tricyclics and SSRIs	Digoxin
	Class Ia antiarrhythmics

covered only by skin and subcutaneous tissue. Confinement to bed is relevant to this. Less often, a foot drop is caused by L5 radiculopathy or polyneuropathy and much less often by sciatic neuropathies, lumbar plexopathies, mononeuritis multiplex or myopathies. Central causes (such as cerebral ischaemia), anterior horn cell diseases, cauda equina compression and muscle dystrophy are rare and usually produce other symptoms.

Reading

Stevens F, Weerkamp NJ, Cals JW. Foot drop. *BMJ* 2015; 350: h1736.

157 Correct Answer: D

Explanation: The clinical history is of value in distinguishing seizure from syncope (see reading below). Light-headedness or blurring of vision before the event are suggestive of syncope; the others make a seizure more likely. Prolonged confusion and aching muscles after the event make seizure more likely, but nausea, vomiting and pallor after the event make syncope more likely. Also, an aura such as a funny smell before the event is more likely for seizure, but nausea, vomiting, abdominal discomfort and feeling of cold sweating are more likely before syncope.

Reading

European Society of Cardiology. 2018 ESC Guidelines for the diagnosis and management of syncope. *European Heart Journal 2018*; 39: 1883–1948.

158 Correct Answer: C

Explanation: According to NICE guidance QS 86, an individualised multifactorial intervention is an intervention with multiple components that aims to address the risk factors for falling that are identified in a person's individual multifactorial assessment, and specific components common in successful multifactorial interventions are strength and balance training, home hazard assessment and intervention, vision assessment and referral, and medication review with modification or withdrawal. However, the following interventions, at the time of publication of this book, have *not been* recommended to address falls risk factors due to insufficient or conflicting evidence, although they may result in other health benefits:

- Low-intensity exercise combined with incontinence programmes group exercise (not individually prescribed)
- Cognitive behavioural interventions
- Referral for correction of visual impairment as a single intervention
- Vitamin D supplementation
- Hip protectors
- Brisk walking

Reading

www.nice.org.uk/guidance/qs86/resources/falls-in-older-people-pdf-2098911933637.

159 Correct Answer: A

Explanation: Lack of participant and intervention provider blinding can be a source of bias. Older people living in care homes are around three times more likely to fall compared with those living in the community. Podiatry interventions reduce falls in older people who live in their own homes, but the evidence is less clear for older people living in care homes. Referral to podiatry services provides reductions in falls, and there is now a strong case for trials of podiatry interventions to reduce falls in care homes.

Reading

Wylie G, Torrens C, Campbell P, et al. Podiatry interventions to prevent falls in older people: A systematic review and meta-analysis. *Age Ageing* 2019; 48 (3): 327–336.

160 Correct Answer: D

Explanation: Proposed mechanisms for the age-related decline in muscle mass and strength include a decrease in physical activity/sedentary lifestyle, undernutrition, hormonal changes, inflammation, oxidative stress and denervation.

Some anatomical and biochemical changes in ageing muscle are discussed in the following sections:

Anatomical Changes

- Reduction in total myofibre number
- Reduced number and size of type II fibres
- Decreased muscle mass and cross-sectional area
- Decrease in number of motor neurons, increase in size of motor units
- Accumulation of noncontractile proteins
- Decreased blood flow

Biochemical Changes

- Decreased myosin heavy chain synthesis
- Increased oxidative stress
- Decline in mitochondrial activity

Reading

Clegg A, Patel H. Frailty and sarcopenia. In *Oxford textbook of medicine* (Sixth edition). Eds. J. Firth, C. Conlon, T. Cox. Oxford, UK: Oxford University Press, 2020. DOI: 10.1093/med/9780198746690.001.0001.

161 Correct Answer: E

Explanation: Current guidance, at the time of publication of this book, is 'Joint Statement on Clinical Selection for Trans-catheter Aortic Valve Implantation (TAVI)', 2017.

None of the existing surgical risk scores has been validated in TAVI, and all omit important clinical variables, including frailty. Work-up investigations have become more streamlined in recent years, and variability exists across centres as to the preferred work-up required. Tests that help determine the suitability and risk for the patient include trans-thoracic echocardiography, which is considered mandatory. Comorbidities that may incline an MDT away from intervention include cognitive impairment, poor mobility, poor respiratory function, poor renal function, severe additional valvular disease (regurgitation or stenosis), impaired right or left ventricular function and severe pulmonary hypertension. TAVI could be considered if there are anatomical limitations to surgery, e.g. extensive aortic calcification ('porcelain aorta') and/or previous chest radiotherapy.

Reading

Joint Statement on clinical selection for Transcatheter Aortic Valve Implantation (TAVI), dated 1/8/2017, on behalf of BCS, SCTS and BCIS. www.bcis.org.uk/wp-content/uploads/2017/08/TAVI-commissioning-statement-final.pdf.

162 Correct Answer: C

Explanation: This question spans across three different clauses of the NICE guidance on transient loss of consciousness: clause 1.1.2.2 for 'red flag' symptoms on a 12 lead ECG, clause 1.1.4.2 for the urgent need for cardiovascular assessment, and clause 1.4.1.1 to consider psychogenic non-epileptic seizures (PNES) or psychogenic pseudosyncope.

According to this guidance, examples of features of these PNES attacks might include the nature of the events changes over time, multiple unexplained physical symptoms and the presence of unusually prolonged events.

Reading

Transient loss of consciousness ('blackouts') in over 16s. Clinical Guideline (CG 109). Published: August 2010. www.nice.org.uk/guidance/cg109.

163 Correct Answer: E

Explanation: PPH has been traditionally defined as a fall in systolic BP of >20 mmHg, or a decrease to <90 mmHg when the pre-prandial BP is <100 mmHg, within two hours of a meal. Current evidence suggests that in most cases there is not a single, or dominant, aetiological factor in PPH. Of the macronutrients, glucose appears to elicit the most rapid decrease in systolic BP in healthy older subjects. It should be recognised that all published studies relating to the clinical manifestations of PPH have substantial limitations, particularly in relation to the size of the cohorts studied, lack of appropriate control subjects, paucity of longitudinal assessments and potential confounders. The effects of withdrawal of antihypertensive therapy in symptomatic PPH have not been formally evaluated yet.

Reading

Trahair LG, Horowitz M, Jones KL. Postprandial hypotension: A systematic review. *J Am Med Dir Assoc* 2014; 15 (6): 394–409.

164 Correct Answer: A

Explanation: This question concerns screening for mobility impairments. An ability to turn without staggering is of note in the 'Timed Up and Go' test. The normal time required to complete the Timed Up and Go test is less than ten seconds. Lower scores on the Tinetti Falls Efficacy Scale indicate greater confidence in walking. The Modified Romberg Test is performed while standing. The Tinetti Falls Efficacy Scale is a ten-item questionnaire. In the Timed Up and Go test, the patient is asked to wear regular footwear and use any customary walking aid.

Reading

Khan RM. Mobility impairment in the elderly. *InnovAiT* 2018; 11 (1): 14–19.

165 Correct Answer: E

Explanation: The diagnosis is vasoglossopharyngeal neuralgia. The history is inconsistent with the other diagnoses. There is no mention of micturition. The history fits the diagnostic criteria provided by the International Association for the Study of Pain. Asystole, convulsions and syncope are associated with vasoglossopharyngeal neuralgia in many patients described in the literature. The trigger zone is recognised late as compared to trigeminal neuralgia; therefore, it may not be found during initial clinical examination. The lack of syncope with lateral neck movements or shaving makes carotid sinus hypersensitivity unlikely. The diagnosis is strictly clinical, as no imaging findings or other testing can reliably link to the syndrome.

Reading

Singh PM, Kaur M, Trikha A. An uncommonly common: Glossopharyngeal neuralgia. *Ann Indian Acad Neurol* 2013; 16 (1): 1–8.

166 Correct Answer: C

Explanation: Unintentional weight loss of ≥ 4.5 kg or ≥ 5% of body mass in the last year (obtained from patient, caregiver or medical records).

Reading

Bieniek J, Wilczyński K, Szewieczek J. Fried frailty phenotype assessment components as applied to geriatric in-patients. *Clin Interv Aging* 2016; 11: 453–459.

Fried LP, Tangen CM, Walston J, et al. Frailty in older adults: Evidence for a phenotype. *J Gerontol a Biol Sci Med Sci* 2001; 56 (3): M146–M156.

Rahman, S. *Living with frailty: From assets to resilience.* Oxford: Routledge, 2018.

167 Correct Answer: C

Explanation: An immune-mediated necrotising myopathy (IMNM) is important to be recognised because it is not a self-limiting adverse effect. Beside discontinuation of the causative statin, an aggressive immunosuppressive therapy is mandatory in IMNM. Therefore, it is important to test for anti-HMGCR antibodies and if necessary perform a muscle biopsy in patients taking statins, presenting with muscle weakness, and CK elevations not improving after discontinuation of the statin. Muscle biopsy is consistent with an IMNM. Due to the clinical and biochemical presentation, the typical muscle biopsy findings and the elevated anti-HMGCR antibodies, the diagnosis of HMGCR antibody-mediated IMNM was presumed. Paraneoplastic antibodies being negative does not suggest dermatomyositis as a diagnosis; the extensive negative viral serology screen argues against viral polymyositis; the negative anti-Jo-1 antibody suggests that antisynthetase syndrome is not the diagnosis; and the muscle biopsy is not suggestive of inclusion body myositis.

Reading

De Cock E, Hannon H, Moerman V, et al. Statin-induced myopathy: A case report. *Eur Heart J Case Rep* December 2018; 2 (4).

Selva-O'Callaghan A, Alvarado-Cardenas M, Pinal-Fernández I, et al. Statin-induced myalgia and myositis: An update on pathogenesis and clinical recommendations. *Expert Rev Clin Immunol* 2018; 14 (3): 215–224.

168 Correct Answer: D

NICE CG161 advises that all patients aged 65 years or older should be regarded as being at risk of falling in hospital. NICE advises against the use of fall risk prediction tools to predict inpatients' risk of falling in hospital. A multifactorial falls risk assessment should be performed by a healthcare professional with appropriate skills and experience, and part of an individualised, multifactorial intervention. Risk factors for falling in hospital that can be treated, improved or managed during their expected stay are listed on p. 9 of NICE CG161 (2020). Various aspects of the history are well known to be relevant to the risk of falling, such as arthritis, Parkinson's disease, incontinence, sensory impairment, cognitive impairment, history of falls or syncope or polypharmacy. Poor footwear or wet surfaces also do not help.

Reading

National Institute for health and Care Excellence. Falls in older people: assessing risk and prevention Clinical guideline [CG161], 12 June 2013. https://www.nice.org.uk/guidance/cg161

169 Correct Answer: E

Explanation: NICE lists glucosamine, chondroitin and acupuncture as interventions that should not be offered in the management of osteoarthritis. Others include rubefacients and intra-articular hyaluronan injections.

NICE does recommend a number of interventions, but the full guidance should be referred to in this context.

Some interventions to note are possible use of the following, described across the whole guidance:

- Local muscle strengthening
- General aerobic fitness
- Weight loss in those who are obese or overweight
- Thermotherapy
- Electrotherapy
- Aids and devices
- Manual therapy
- Topical NSAIDs (particularly in knee or hand osteoarthritis)
- Topical capsaicin
- Intra-articular corticosteroid injections
- Surgical options (only once non-surgical interventions have been explored)

Clause 1.5.2 specifically addresses oral analgesics.

Reading

National Institute for Health and Care Excellence. Osteoarthritis: Care and management. Clinical Guideline [CG177], February 2014. www.nice. org.uk/guidance/cg177/chapter/1-recommendations.

170 Correct Answer: D

Explanation: This question is testing a candidate's ability to diagnose reflex syncope based on the clinical assessment. Reflex syncope, also called neural-mediated syncope, refers to situations in which reflexes normally involved in blood pressure and heart rate control become acutely inappropriate, leading to a sudden drop in cerebral blood perfusion. According to NICE guidance; do not offer a tilt test to people who have a diagnosis of vasovagal syncope on initial assessment; for people with suspected vasovagal syncope with recurrent episodes of transient loss of consciousness adversely affecting their quality of life or representing a high risk of injury, consider a tilt test only to assess whether the syncope is accompanied by a severe cardioinhibitory response (usually asystole).

Reading

Transient loss of consciousness ('blackouts') in over 16s. Clinical Guideline [CG109]. Published: 25 August 2010 Last updated: 1 September 2014. www.nice.org.uk/guidance/cg109.

171 Correct Answer: D

Explanation: A sudden onset of limb weakness and altered neurology in a person with atrial fibrillation is most likely to be due to embolic phenomena. All the other diagnoses on the list would present with neurological symptoms which progress over days to weeks. An adverse effect from amoxicillin use is unlikely to present this way. Other differentials could potentially include tumour or bleed, and an urgent MRI is indicated to rule out a compressive lesion. However, given the very sudden onset and a likely source of embolism, spinal cord infarction is first on the list of differentials. Risk factors for vascular cord syndromes include diabetes hypertension and atrial fibrillation. Symptoms, which generally appear within minutes or a few hours of the infarction, may include intermittent sharp or burning back pain, aching pain down through the legs, weakness in the legs, paralysis, loss of deep tendon reflexes, loss of pain and temperature sensation, and incontinence.

Reading

Spinal Cord Infarction Information Page, NINDS. www.ninds.nih.gov/disorders/all-disorders/spinal-cord-infarction-information-page.

7

Geriatric Assessment

> **LEARNING OBJECTIVE:**
>
> Factors affecting health status and measurement of health status.

Areas to cover are:

- An ability to perfórm a comprehensive geriatric assessment (CGA), which includes physical, functional, social, environmental, psychological and spiritual concerns.
- Current evidence base for CGA.
- Non-specific acute presentations seen in older patients.
- Assessment of multimorbidity and polypharmacy (including principles of medicines reconciliation and deprescribing).
- Assessment of frailty (including frailty scales).
- Factors influencing health status in older people.
- Measuring health status and outcome.
- Safeguarding legislation and actions needed when caring for vulnerable adults.

Questions

Question 172

When defining frailty using the Fried model, which one of the following criteria should be considered?

A. polypharmacy

B. sensory impairment (sight or hearing)

C. performance on 'Timed Up and Go' test

D. two or more falls within the last year

E. unintentional weight loss

Question 173

A 91-year-old woman is referred to the geriatrics outpatient clinic by her GP, who is concerned that her functional level is declining. Over the last year she has become unable to manage her housework, and carers now assist her with washing and dressing. She has a past medical history of biventricular cardiac failure and urinary incontinence. You decided to apply a screening tool to identify frailty. Which of the following is assessed in the PRISMA-7 questionnaire?

A. age

B. gait speed

C. grip strength

D. mood

E. sleep

Question 174

You see an 87-year-old woman in the older persons' assessment clinic who has fallen over her front room rug. It is intended that the five domains are completed in a 'comprehensive geriatric assessment'. The carer has not been contacted yet. What is the next best step?

A. contacting her carer

B. creation of a problem list

C. intervention

D. personalised care planning

E. regular planned review

Question 175

Which of the following can maximise the impact of a comprehensive geriatric assessment?

A. clear barriers in use of information

B. confidential documentation held only by clinicians

C. development of multi-professional teams and regular multidisciplinary team reviews

D. maintaining a hierarchy between medical and social care staff

E. the comprehensive geriatric assessment must be completed first by a junior doctor

Question 176

Which of the following statements is true about the functional and social assessment during a comprehensive geriatric assessment process?

A. most healthcare consultations are done at the patient's home

B. most healthcare consultations are done with informal carers present

C. one of the main problems with the Barthel Index is the 'ceiling effect'

D. 'step changes' in function are of little relevance to goal setting

E. the 'Timed Up and Go' test is only a test of physical ability

Question 177

Which of the following scales defines frailty as the presence of three of the following five variables: unexplained weight loss, low grip strength, slow walking, self-reported exhaustion and low physical activity?

A. Canadian Study of Health and Aging Clinical Frailty Scale

B. Fried's 'Phenotypic frailty' scale

C. Identification of Seniors at Risk

D. Stable gait, Unstable gait, Help to walk or Bedridden scale

E. Triage Risk Screening Tool

Question 178

The Malnutrition Universal Screening Tool (MUST) is used to identify adults who are malnourished, at risk of malnutrition (undernutrition) or obese. You learn that an 82-year-old care home resident is found to have a MUST score of 2. What is the most appropriate next step?

A. do nothing

B. document dietary intake for three days

C. refer to dietitian or nutritional support team or implement local policy

D. repeat screening monthly

E. repeat screening weekly

Question 179

Which of the following is an index, not criteria, to assess inappropriate prescribing in older patients?

A. Assessment of Underutilisation of Medication

B. Beers

C. McLeod

D. START

E. STOPP

Question 180

According to the current European Working Group on Sarcopenia in Older People (EWGSOP2) criteria, sarcopenia is most likely to be present in which of the following situations?

A. 400 m walk test time greater than four minutes

B. Grip strength less than 27 kg for men and women

C. Short Physical Performance Battery score 10 or more

D. Timed Up and Go test 20 seconds or more

E. Walking speed, one metre per second or slower

Question 181

How many long-term health conditions fulfil the National Institute for Health and Care Excellence definition of multimorbidity?

A. two or more

B. three or more

C. four or more

D. five or more

E. six or more

Question 182

Which statement about the assessment of frailty is correct?

A. a score >4 on PRISMA-7 identifies frailty

B. polypharmacy is considered when the patient is taking eight or more medications

C. slow walking speed is considered less than 0.6 m/s

D. the Groningen Frailty Indicator questionnaire is a 15-item frailty questionnaire that is suitable for postal completion. A score of more than four indicates the possible presence of moderate to severe frailty

E. the Timed Up and Go test involves walking a distance of 4 metres

Question 183

Current European guidelines suggest that the SARC-F test can be used as a screening tool to help detect people with sarcopenia. Regarding the SARC-F test, which of the following statements is correct?

A. a score of zero suggests severe sarcopenia

B. assessment involves carrying a 10 kg weight across a room

C. it can include CT scan measurements of psoas muscle diameter, when available

D. it includes a measure of gait speed

E. it includes asking about number of falls in the last year

Answers for Chapter 7

172 Correct Answer: E

Explanation: Fried identified the frailty phenotype, and it is defined as having three or more of the following five criteria: unintentional weight loss, exhaustion, muscle weakness, slowness while walking and low levels of activity. The Fried model focuses solely on physical attributes of frailty and possibly is an incomplete model in that it does not address cognitive aspects or chronic conditions, which might be associated with frailty.

Reading

Clegg A, Young J, Iliffe S, et al. Frailty in elderly people. *Lancet* 2013; 381 (9868): 752–762.

Fried LP, Tangen CM, Walston J, et al. Frailty in older adults: Evidence for a phenotype. *J Gerontol A Biol Sci Med Sci* 2001; 56 (3): M146–M156.

Fried LP, Xue QL, Cappola AR, Ferrucci L, Chaves P, Varadhan R, Guralnik JM, Leng SX, Semba RD, Walston JD, Blaum CS, Bandeen-Roche K. Nonlinear multisystem physiological dysregulation associated with frailty in older women: Implications for etiology and treatment. *J Gerontol A Biol Sci Med Sci* 2009; 64(10): 1049–1057.

173 Correct Answer: A

Explanation: In hospital outpatient settings, the PRISMA-7 questionnaire is one of the tools recommended to screen for frailty by NICE and the BGS. It includes the following questions:

- Are you more than 85 years old?
- Are you male?
- In general, do you have any health problems that require you to limit your activities?
- Do you need someone to help you on a regular basis?
- In general, do you have any health problems that require you to stay at home?
- In case of need, can you count on someone close to you?
- Do you regularly use a stick, walker or wheelchair to get about?

Reading

PRISMA7 questionnaire. www.hcpa.info/wp-content/uploads/2018/06/PRISMA-Frailty-Assessment-1.pdf.

174 Correct Answer: A

Explanation: The key issue is the collaboration between patient/family/carers and the various members of the team throughout the process. The next best step is the creation of a problem list. It will then accommodate the individual's own personal goals before documenting interventions and overall management strategies, as well as who will deliver these, i.e. a comprehensive care plan.

Reading

British Geriatrics Society. CGA in Primary Care Settings: The elements of the CGA process. www.bgs.org.uk/resources/2-cga-in-primary-care-settings-the-elements-of-the-cga-process.

175 Correct Answer: C

Explanation: Key processes and structures which support implementation and maximise the impact of using comprehensive geriatric assessment:

- Development of multi-professional teams.
- Clear identification of a joint core level of competence in assessment between health and social care practitioners.
- Referrals to other practitioners, external to the team, in the development of a comprehensive care plan.
- Single patient-held documentation.
- Mechanisms for information sharing.
- Regular multidisciplinary team review meetings to share knowledge and develop team working.
- Access to joint health and social care funding.
- Main beneficiaries include older hospital inpatients.

Reading

British Geriatrics Society. CGA in Primary Care Settings: The elements of the CGA process. www. bgs.org.uk/resources/2-cga-in-primary-care-settings-the-elements-of-the-cga-process.

Chadborn NH, Goodman C, Zubair M, Sousa L, Gladman JRF, Dening T, Gordon AL. Rôle of comprehensive geriatric assessment in healthcare of older people in UK care homes: Realist review. *BMJ Open* 8 April 2019; 9(4): e026921.

Parker SG, McCue P, Phelps K, McCleod A, Arora S, Nockels K, Kennedy S, Roberts H, Conroy S. What is comprehensive geriatric assessment (CGA)? An umbrella review. *Age Ageing* 1 January 2018ary; 47(1): 149–155.

176 Correct Answer: C

Explanation: One of the problems with Barthel is its so-called ceiling effect. This means that because it measures very basic function in terms of daily life, one can score quite well on the Barthel and yet still be pretty dependent on others for daily life—for example cooking, laundry, cleaning and shopping. The other statements are not true. The Timed Up and Go test can also be a good indicator of overall function, combining an assessment of physical ability—being able to indeed 'get up and go'—and a test of cognition relating specifically to following instructions and carrying them out successfully. Evidence shows us that intervening at these times of step changes can help to slow a loss of function, and with the right therapies, exercise and goal setting, we can see some reversal and ultimately the patient may regain some physical function. Most healthcare consultations are done out of the patient's home and without the next of kin or informal carers present.

Reading

British Geriatrics Society. CGA in Primary Care Settings: Functional and social assessment. www. bgs.org.uk/resources/4-cga-in-primary-care-settings-functional-and-social-assessment.

177 Correct Answer: B

Explanation: Fried's   'phenotypic frailty' scale, based on data from the Cardiovascular Health Study, defines frailty as the presence of three of the following five variables: unexplained weight loss, low grip strength, slow walking, self-reported exhaustion and low physical activity.

Reading

Lewis ET, Dent E, Alkhouri H, et al. Which frailty scale for patients admitted via emergency department? A cohort study. *Arch Gerontol Geriatr* 2019; 80: 104–114.

178 Correct Answer: C

Explanation:

Score 0—Low Risk
- Routine clinical care
- Repeat screening
- Hospital—weekly
- Care Home—monthly

Score 1—Medium Risk
- Observe
- Document dietary intake for three days
- If adequate—little concern and repeat screening
- Hospital—weekly
- Care Home—at least monthly
- If inadequate—clinical concern—follow local policy, set goals, improve and increase overall nutritional intake, monitor and review care plan regularly

Score 2 or more—High Risk
- Treat
- Refer to dietitian or nutritional support team or implement local policy
- Set goals, improve and increase overall nutritional intake

- Monitor and review care plan
- Hospital—weekly
- Care Home—monthly

Reading

Malnutrition Universal Screening Tool. www.bapen. org.uk/pdfs/must/must_full.pdf.

179 Correct Answer: A

Explanation: Assessment of Underutilisation of Medication is an index. The rest are criteria.

Reading

Cooper JA, Cadogan CA, Patterson SM, et al. Interventions to improve the appropriate use of polypharmacy in older people: A Cochrane systematic review. *BMJ Open* 2015; 5: e009235.

180 Correct Answer: D

Explanation: Grip strength <27 kg for men and <16 kg for women are used to define low muscle strength. Values <20 kg for men and <15 kg for women are used to define low muscle quantity or quality. The following findings also suggest sarcopenia:

- Gait speed 0.8 m/s or slower
- Short Physical Performance Battery (SPPB), score 8 or less
- Timed Up and Go test, 20 seconds or more
- 400 m walking test 6 min or more

SPPB includes timed measures of balance when standing, walking speed and standing up from a chair. Scores range from 0 to 12 with lower scores suggesting greater impairment. Probable sarcopenia is identified by low muscle strength. Sarcopenia is diagnosed when both low muscle strength and reduced muscle quantity or quality are demonstrated. If low physical performance is also present, then the sarcopenia is classified as severe.

Reading

Cruz-Jentoft AJ, Bahat G, Bauer J, et al. Sarcopenia: Revised European consensus on definition and diagnosis. *Age Ageing* 2019; 48: 16–31.

181 Correct Answer: A

Explanation: The NICE guideline on multimorbidity explains that multimorbidity refers to the presence of two or more long-term health conditions, which can include defined physical and mental health conditions such as diabetes or schizophrenia, ongoing conditions such as learning disability, symptom complexes such as frailty or chronic pain, sensory impairment such as sight or hearing loss and alcohol and substance misuse.

Reading

National Institute for Health and Care Excellence. Multimorbidity and polypharmacy. 2017. www. nice.org.uk/guidance/ktt18.

182 Correct Answer: D

Explanation: The PRISMA-7 questionnaire is a seven-item questionnaire to identify disability that has been used in earlier frailty studies and is also suitable for postal completion. A score of >3 is considered to identify frailty. The Timed Up and Go test measures, in seconds, the time taken to stand up from a standard chair, walk a distance of 3 metres, turn, walk back to the chair and sit down. Gait speed is usually measured in m/s and has been recorded over distances ranging from 2.4 m to 6 m in research studies. In this study, gait speed was recorded over a 4 m distance. A slow walking speed (less than 0.8 m/s or taking more than 5 secs to walk 4 m); the PRISMA-7 questionnaire and the Timed Up and Go test (with a cut-off score of 10 secs) had very good sensitivity but only moderate specificity for identifying frailty. 'Self-reported health' is assessed with the question, 'How would you rate your health on a scale of 0–10?'. A cut-off of <6 is used to identify frailty. A GP can assess participants as frail or not frail based on a clinical assessment. For multiple medications (polypharmacy), frailty is deemed present if the person takes five or more medications. The Groningen Frailty Indicator questionnaire is a 15-item frailty questionnaire that is suitable for postal completion. A score of >4 indicates the possible presence of moderate to severe frailty.

Reading

British Geriatrics Society. Recognising frailty. www. bgs.org.uk/resources/recognising-frailty.

183 Correct Answer: E

Explanation: SARC-F is a screening test used to help detect sarcopenia. It has five components: strength (perceived difficulty carrying 5 kg), walking across a room, transferring from chair or bed, climbing a flight of stairs and falls in the last year. Scores range from 0 to 10 (i.e. 0–2 points for each component; 0 = no impairment, 1 = mild impairment, 2 = severe impairment/unable; 0 = best to 10 = worst). A score of 4 or more suggests sarcopenia may be present.

Reading

Malmstrom TK, Miller DK, Simonsick EM, et al. SARC-F: A symptom score to predict persons with sarcopenia at risk for poor functional outcomes. *J Cachexia Sarcopenia Muscle* 2016; 7: 28–36.

8

Surgical Liaison

LEARNING OBJECTIVE:

To know how to 'risk assess', optimise and manage the older elective and emergency surgical patient throughout all parts of the surgical pathway.

Areas to cover are:

- Demographics and political landscape relevant to the older surgical patient.
- 'Fitness for surgery'.
- Clinical assessment with appropriate use of investigations and tools to risk assess for perioperative morbidity and mortality.
- Perioperative management of common comorbid conditions (pain, fluid balance, heart failure, venous thromboembolism, pneumonia and acute kidney injury).
- Perioperative effects and risks of surgery and anaesthesia on older people, including depending on patient factors (e.g. frailty and multimorbidity) and surgical factors (e.g. type of surgery and anaesthesia).
- National audits to improve quality of care.
- Management of surgical issues and complications, e.g. 'failure to thrive', sepsis, wound infections, pain, arrhythmias, heart failure, renal injury, pain control, tissue viability, wound management, indications for repeat X-ray, non-union.

- Use of interdisciplinary and cross-speciality interventions to improve postoperative outcome (e.g. therapy delivered 'prehabilitation').
- Use of interventions to improve post-operative outcome (e.g. multimodal prehabilitation).
- Service development.

Questions

Question 184

The concept of 'prehabilitation' for older people prior to having major surgical procedures has recently been gaining attention. Which of the following statements is most likely to be correct?

A. a diet containing at least 1 g per kg of protein is required to address preoperative malnutrition

B. high-intensity interval training (HIIT) exercise methods should be avoided in people due to have cardiovascular surgical procedures

C. psychological support to address anxiety and depression has been shown to improve surgical outcomes

D. reducing alcohol intake to 14 units per week or less reduces the incidence of post-operative complications

E. smoking cessation one to two weeks prior to surgery has been shown to reduce post-operative complications

Question 185

These days, many people with dementia undergo surgical procedures. You are asked to help create joint management guidelines for this patient group for your hospital. Which of the following statements is most likely to be correct for people with dementia?

A. donepezil, whenever possible, should be discontinued 48 hours prior to elective surgery

B. memantine increases the risk of neurocognitive toxicity with ketamine

C. post-operative cognitive decline is defined as occurring within 30 days of a surgical procedure

D. regional anaesthesia use lowers the risk of post-operative delirium

E. volatile anaesthetic agents are usually preferred to propofol

Question 186

An 82-year-old needs an effective nerve block for reducing pain after a hip fracture. What is the block of choice?

A. combined nerve blocks

B. epidural

C. fascia-iliaca block

D. femoral nerve block

E. psoas compartment block

Question 187

Which one of the following statements concerning emergency laparotomy in older surgical patients is true?

A. at present, geriatric liaison care is only available for around 20%–25% of older surgical patients and does not always include the emergency surgical patient

B. frailty is not associated with increased mortality or increased length of stay for patients who survive surgery

C. prehabilitation is a useful intervention in emergency operations

D. short-term mortality in older patients following emergency surgery is about 10% one year after surgery

E. the risk prediction tool PPOSSUM is useful in surgical liaison for older people with frailty

Question 188

An 82-year-old man presented after an episode of vasovagal syncope with loss of consciousness, which resulted in him hitting his head on the coffee table. His medication included clopidogrel, bisoprolol and simvastatin. On examination, his temperature was 38.0°C. He had a cut on left scalp with bloodstains over his shirt; he also had severe bruising on his abdomen and was tender in the left hypochondrium.

What is the most appropriate next investigation?

A. CT scan of abdomen

B. lower gastrointestinal endoscopy

C. MR scan of brain

D. upper gastrointestinal endoscopy

E. X-ray of abdomen

TABLE 8.1

Investigations.

Haemoglobin	86 g/L (130–170)
MCV	90 fL (80–96)
Platelet count	Normal
CT head	Subarachnoid bleeding over the convexity of the left frontoparietal lobe but no skull fracture

Answers for Chapter 8

184 Correct Answer: D

Explanation: Reducing alcohol intake, when relevant, to within recommended levels (i.e. 14 units per week or less) also reduces the incidence of post-operative complications. Smoking cessation four to six weeks prior to surgery has been shown to reduce post-operative complications, including pneumonia, myocardial ischaemia and impaired wound healing. High-intensity interval training may be a more time-efficient way to improve aerobic capacity and appears to be safe even in people awaiting vascular surgery. Ideally, muscle mass would also be increased with resistance training because low muscle mass is associated with worse outcomes. Inspiratory muscle training can also be used to target respiratory muscle strength and reduce the risk of post-operative pneumonia. An adapted version of the Malnutrition Universal Screening Tool (MUST) can be used to assess preoperative nutritional status. A protein intake of 1.5 to 2 g/kg is recommended to address preoperative malnutrition, especially when aiming to improve muscle mass.

Reading

Durrand J, Singh S, Danjoux G. Prehabilitation. *Clin Med* 2019; 6: 458–464.

185 Correct Answer: B

Explanation: Memantine can enhance the central nervous system toxicity of ketamine.

A discussion around the neurocognitive risks of surgery and anaesthesia should be part of the consent process for older patients, but there is currently much uncertainty. In practice, it can be difficult to clinically distinguish pre-existing cognitive changes, post-operative delirium and post-operative cognitive decline (defined as occurring between seven days and one year of surgery). Anticholinergic adverse effects are possible from a wide range of anaesthetic and analgesic drugs. Currently there is no strong evidence that postoperative delirium or mortality rates differ between general and regional anaesthesia use.

Reading

White S, Griffiths R, Baxter M, et al. Guidelines for the peri-operative care of people with dementia. *Anaesthesia* 2019; 74: 357–372.

186 Correct Answer: C

Explanation: Various modalities of regional nerve blockade, including epidural, fascia-iliaca block, femoral nerve block, psoas compartment block and combined nerve blocks, have all been shown to be effective in rapidly reducing acute pain following a hip fracture. When used, they reduce the need for breakthrough analgesia and opiates, but a fascia-iliaca block may well be the block of choice, given that it has been shown that it can be administered both safely and rapidly under ultrasound guidance in the emergency department and acute ward setting.

Reading

Parke S, Eaves C, Dimond S, et al. Perioperative optimization of hip fracture patients. *Orthopaedic and Trauma* 2020; 34: 80–88.

187 Correct Answer: A

Explanation: At present, geriatric liaison care is only available for 23% of older surgical patients and does not always include the emergency surgical patient.

Prehabilitation or 'prehab' is currently gaining popularity. Optimising patients, particularly in older age groups, before the marathon of elective surgery is gaining momentum worldwide. Risk prediction tools exist and are commonly used. For older patients who survive surgery, frailty is associated with worse surgical outcomes: increased mortality, prolonged hospital stay, complications and an increased level of social care provision on discharge from hospital.

Reading

McCarthy K, Hewitt J. Special needs of frail people undergoing emergency laparotomy surgery. *Age Ageing* 2020; 49 (4): 540–543.

188 Correct Answer: A

Explanation: The degree of anaemia is not explained by a small traumatic subarachnoid haemorrhage. The patient has sustained a left upper abdominal injury, so a splenic injury should be suspected, which is a surgical emergency.

9

Intermediate Care and Long-Term Care

> **LEARNING OBJECTIVE:**
>
> To have the knowledge and skills required to assess a patient's suitability for and deliver care to older people within intermediate care and long-term care settings, working with multidisciplinary teams, primary care and local authority colleagues to achieve this.

Areas to cover are:

- The significance of patients with frailty in these services.
- Models of intermediate care/community geriatrics, including evolving rôle of day hospital.
- Opportunities provided by assistive technologies, e.g. monitoring devices, technology-assisted living.
- Current evidence base for intermediate and community care.
- Current national publications regarding intermediate care.
- Rôle of commissioning in services for older people.
- Regulation regarding medicine administration in care homes.
- Models of medical care for care home patients, including knowledge of evidence base.
- Knowledge of pressure-relieving and other specialist equipment and their uses.
- Understanding of the various agencies involved in community care.

- Relevant national publications, including guidelines on continuing healthcare.
- Relevant national publications, including guidelines on respite care.
- Importance of medicines optimisation.
- Understanding of care home structures, regulation and inspection.
- Appropriate pharmacological and non-pharmacological interventions.
- 'Smart homes'.

Questions

Question 189

A 92-year-old woman has decided to move into a care home due to increased physical care needs. She does not have cognitive impairment and is concerned that all the other residents will be cognitively impaired, reducing her prospects of having meaningful interactions with them. What is the closest current estimate to the proportion of people in care homes in the UK who are known to have cognitive impairment?

A. 20%

B. 40%

C. 60%

D. 80%

E. 100%

Question 190

High-quality care in care homes would be best characterised by which one of the following metrics?

A. annual medication review

B. fewer hospital admissions

C. greater rate of antipsychotic drug use

D. low rates of advance care planning

E. reactive approach to problems

Question 191

The wife of a 79-year-old man with dementia reports increasing stress relating to providing care for her husband at home. They are both keen to avoid a permanent care home placement if possible. The concept of respite care has been discussed. Which of the following statements is most likely to be true regarding respite care for people with dementia?

A. carer sleep quality is improved during a period of residential care for the person with dementia

B. day care delays the time to care home admission

C. respite care within the person's own home is usually unhelpful

D. temporary residential care reduces carer stress immediately after the placement period

E. the recipient's sleep quality is likely to improve during a period of temporary residential care

Question 192

Which of the following is typically true for high-quality intermediate care services for older people with frailty?

A. a three-month duration is typical

B. it should start within two days of a referral being made to the service

C. risk avoidance should underpin decisions

D. service provision is entirely provided within a care home or community hospital setting

E. unsuitable for people with moderate to severe dementia

Question 193

Approximately what proportion of emergency hospital bed days are occupied by residents of care homes in the UK?

A. 4%

B. 8%

C. 12%

D. 16%

E. 20%

Question 194

Which of the following statements is correct regarding medication use in care homes in the UK?

A. care home staff should contact the relevant GP for advice if a resident should decline to take a dose of a prescribed medication

B. decisions about medicines optimisation should be made by the resident's doctor and next of kin

C. residents should be supported to self-administer medications

D. suspected drug adverse reactions should be discussed at six-monthly medication reviews

E. there is no requirement to record medication-related safety events that do not result in injury

Question 195

A good practice guidance from the Royal Pharmaceutical Society provides four guiding principles for medicines optimisation that will help all healthcare professionals to support patients to get the best outcomes from their medications. A patient recently home from hospital kept missing his dose of antipsychotic medicine because it was labelled 'Take one tablet in the morning'. He frequently woke after midday. What principle does this vignette illustrate?

A. principle 1. Aim to understand the patient's experience

B. principle 2. Evidence-based choice of medicines

C. principle 3. Ensure medicines use is as safe as possible

D. principle 4. Make medicines optimisation part of routine practice

E. none of principles 1–4

Question 196

Which of the following groups of people are unlikely to be appropriate for intermediate care as a first option?

A. care home residents

B. patients intended for reablement within home care

C. patients living in temporary accommodation

D. patients with dementia

E. prisoners

Question 197

Rakesh, a 76-year-old retired solicitor, has recently had a landline phone and broadband connection installed. Two of his cousins work in information technology in Bangalore; they organised the connection, set up an email account, taught Rakesh how to use his tablet, laptop and various videoconferencing apps, and are available to fix any problems. His tablet was purchased by a friend and given to him while he was on the stroke unit. He has hundreds of apps on it freely downloaded off the internet and appears to use them effectively; many apps are games for leisure, but some are for remote communication, and he also has exercise video apps for his arms and legs. What aspect of assistive technology does this vignette illustrate?

A. bricolage

B. capability

C. materiality

D. smart homes

E. telemonitoring

Question 198

Regulators use certain features as metrics to judge the quality of care homes. Which of the following is usually held as important in such regulation?

A. early notice period of consumer care contract

B. good reputation

C. quality of Wi-Fi coverage

D. value for money

E. well-led

Question 199

In the past decades, many studies evaluated the predictors of institutionalisation for older people. Which of the following has consistently had strong evidence for prediction of institutionalisation?

A. arthritis

B. dementia

C. hypertension

D. incontinence

E. respiratory diseases

Question 200

A daughter of a man with dementia attends his GP practice. He has been falling over due to forgetting to use his four-wheeled walking frame. This mainly occurs at night when he needs to go to the toilet. The patient is confused but has no behavioural problems. He lives alone (his daughter is visiting from Scotland) and has carers attending twice a day to assist with meals and getting dressed. He also forgot to turn off the cooker last week. He has already attended falls clinic and the old age psychiatry clinic; both report a general decline in this cognitive function. His daughter wants to make plans for her father to be safe. He has indicated that he would like to go into a care home. What do you think is the best option for this patient?

A. dementia specialist care home placement

B. nursing home placement

C. remain at home and reassess in one year

D. residential home placement

E. respite care

Question 201

In the 'Silver Book' of quality care for older people with urgent and emergency care needs, which of the following is a recommendation on discharge planning?

A. a dipstick of the urine must be performed

B. carers and families should be always involved in the decision-making process around assessment and management of future care

C. care home providers should be treated as equal partners in the planning and commissioning of care

D. information should not be shared between services because of confidentiality

E. there is no requirement to consult older people and carers about their preference for discharge destinations

Answers to Chapter 9

189 Correct Answer: D

Explanation: Currently over 400,000 people, and around 16% of people aged over 85, live in care homes in the UK. It is estimated that 75%–80% of care home residents have cognitive impairment.

Reading

British Geriatrics Society. Effective healthcare for older people living in care homes: Guidance on commissioning and providing healthcare services across the UK. 2016. www.bgs.org.uk/resources/effective-healthcare-for-older-people-living-in-care-homes.

190 Correct Answer: B

Explanation: A proactive approach to care should be adopted, rather than a reactive one, aiming to seek potential future problems before they occur. Six-monthly medication reviews are recommended. Lower rates of antipsychotic drug use, lower rates of hospital admission and higher rates of advance care planning are associated with better care quality.

Reading

British Geriatrics Society. Effective healthcare for older people living in care homes: Guidance on commissioning and providing healthcare services across the UK. 2016. www.bgs.org.uk/resources/effective-healthcare-for-older-people-living-in-care-homes.

191 Correct Answer: A

Explanation: Temporary residential care in a care home results in improved carer sleep quality during, but increased burden and stress immediately after, the respite period. Recipients' sleep quality usually declines during this type of respite. They also need to adapt to two changes in environment and routine (admission and discharge home). In-home respite care has only limited data so far, but a positive impact has been suggested.

Respite care for people with dementia can help their carer to continue delivering a challenging rôle by reducing stress and overburden. It can be delivered as day care or residential care either within their own home or in a care home setting. Barriers can include carer guilt, recipient acceptance, financial cost and availability. Day care has been shown to have positive outcomes for recipients and carers, including reduced burden and reduced behavioural problems. However, studies have suggested that its use may reduce the time to care home placement.

Reading

Vandepitte S, Van Den Noortgate N, Putman K, et al. Effectiveness of respite care in supporting informal caregivers of persons with dementia: A systematic review. *Int J Geriatr Psychiatry* 2016; 31: 1277–1288.

192 Correct Answer: B

Explanation: Intermediate care should start within two days of a referral being made. Episodes of intermediate care typically last less than six weeks. Services should not exclude people with specific conditions, such as dementia, or those who live in care homes. It can be provided through extra support within the recipient's own home (e.g. crisis support) or in a bed-based capacity within a specific unit. Positive risk taking is standard practice. This balances the potential benefits of risk-taking (e.g. independence) against possible negative effects (e.g. falls).

Reading

National Institute for Health and Care Excellence. Intermediate care including reablement. 2017. www.nice.org.uk/guidance/ng74.

193 Correct Answer: B

Explanation: It is estimated that 7.7% of emergency hospital bed days are occupied by care home residents. Once admitted, the average length of stay is 8.9 days for residential care home residents and 7.4 days for those who live in nursing homes.

Reading

Wolters A, Santos F, Lloyd T, et al. Emergency admissions to hospital from care homes: How often and what for? The Health Foundation, 2019. www.health.org.uk/publications/reports/emergency-admissions-to-hospital-from-care-homes.

194 Correct Answer: C

Explanation: Care home residents have the same rights to be involved in healthcare decisions as people who do not reside in care homes. If a medication is declined, the circumstances and reason (if known) should be recorded. If the resident consents, ongoing refusal can be reported to the prescribing team so that supply can be discontinued (starting with the assumption that the resident has capacity to make informed decisions). Residents should, wherever possible, be involved in medicines optimisation decisions. They should also be supported to self-administer where possible. Suspected adverse drug reactions should be reported immediately, including to out-of-hours services when relevant. All medication-related safety events should be recorded irrespective of harm, including near misses.

Reading

National Institute for Health and Care Excellence. Managing medicines in care homes. 2014. ww.nice. org.uk/guidance/sc1.

195 Correct Answer: A

Explanation: Principle 1: to promote this principle. . .

- Patients are more engaged, understand more about their medicines and are able to make choices, including choices about prevention and healthy living.
- Patients' beliefs and preference about medicines are understood to enable a shared decision about treatment.
- Patients are able to take/use their medicines as agreed.
- Patients feel confident enough to share openly their experiences of taking or not taking medicines, their views about what medicines mean to them, and how medicines impact on their daily life.

Reading

Royal Pharmaceutical Society. Medicines optimisation: Helping patients to make the most of medicines. Good practice guidance for healthcare professionals in England. 2013. www.rpharms.com/Portals/0/RPS%20document%20library/Open%20access/Policy/helping-patients-make-the-most-of-their-medicines.pdf.

196 Correct Answer: C

Explanation: This question examines interpretation of the NICE guidance on intermediate care (2017) found in clauses 1.3.2 and 1.4.2, which outline which patients should not be excluded from intermediate care and patients to whom reablement should be offered as a first option.

Reading

National Institute for Health and Care Excellence. Intermediate care including reablement. 2017. www.nice.org.uk/guidance/ng74.

197 Correct Answer: A

Explanation: Essential requirements for the 'bricoleur' rôle include a detailed understanding of participants' needs and wishes, an ability to match these needs to technologies available in the home or obtainable and affordable outside it, some technical ability and a willingness and capacity to revisit the home setting to adjust the technology when needed. Telemonitoring encompasses the use of audio, video and other telecommunication technologies to monitor patient status at a distance. Smart-home technologies include different types of active and passive sensors, monitoring devices, robotics and environmental control systems.

Reading

Greenhalgh T, Wherton J, Sugarhood P, et al. What matters to older people with assisted living needs? A phenomenological analysis of the use and non-use of telehealth and telecare. *Soc Sci Med* 2013; 93: 86–94.

198 Correct Answer: E

Explanation: For example, the function of the Care Quality Commission is to monitor and inspect health and adult social care services such as local care homes, GP practices and hospitals. Key metrics for them include safety, responsiveness to people's needs, effectiveness, being well-led and caring.

Reading

'What can you expect from a good care home?', Care Quality Commission. www.cqc.org.uk/help-advice/what-expect-good-care-services/what-can-you-expect-good-care-home.

199 Correct Answer: B

Explanation: Dementia is considered the most common cause for nursing home placement. Studies showed the risk increasing up to 17-fold, highlighting the overwhelming impact of dementia on nursing home placement, caused by the rapid decrease of an individual's ability to live independently, which is again caused by increasing cognitive impairment and related disabilities in ADL and IADL.

Reading

Luppa M, Luck T, Weyerer S, et al. Prediction of institutionalization in the elderly: A systematic review. *Age Ageing* 2010; 39 (1): 31–38.

200 Correct Answer: D

Explanation: Residential home placement would be the best option for this patient. His main issue is safety (falls, leaving on the cooker). The patient is able to self-care with personal hygiene—he just needs assistance with dressing and meals. He does not need nursing care. The patient has no behavioural difficulties, therefore an 'elderly mentally infirm' (EMI) placement would be inappropriate at this stage. Respite care is only a short-term option; it is unlikely that the patient's condition will improve. Whilst the majority of older adults live in their own home, the patient is at risk of injuring himself or causing a house explosion if he remains at home for much longer.

Reading

Advising older people about their housing choices in later life: A self training module for advisers. www.housingcare.org/downloads/kbase/3126.pdf.

201 Correct Answer: C

Explanation: The original 'Silver Book' was published by the British Geriatrics Society. It recommends ways in which emergency admissions can be reduced and the experience of those admitted improved. Where appropriate, carers and families should be involved in the decision-making process around the assessment and management of future care. Adequate and timely information must be shared between services whenever there is a transfer of care. Older people should only be discharged from hospital with adequate support and with respect for their preferences. The 'Silver Book' was updated by the British Geriatrics Society in 2021.

Reading

BGS Silver book II, 21 February 2021. https://www.bgs.org.uk/resources/resource-series/silver-book-ii.

10

Nutrition

LEARNING OBJECTIVE:

To know how to assess the nutritional status of older people across various care settings and in conjunction with other relevant health professionals to be able to devise an appropriate nutritional support strategy for patients.

Areas to cover are:

- Basic physiology of the digestive system.
- Epidemiology of nutrition and malnutrition.
- Nutritional assessment, including assessment tools such as the Malnutrition Universal Screening Tool (MUST).
- Risk factors and poor nutrition.
- Investigation for patients with malabsorption.
- Provision of strategies to enhance nutrition.
- Nutritional support including indications, delivery routes (oral, nasogastric, including 'nasal bridles', gastrostomy, parenteral) and potential problems.
- Multidisciplinary team working (dietician, nutrition support team, gastroenterologist).
- Nutritional requirements of older adults (malabsorption states in stroke and other neurological causes of dysphagia, dementia and delirium, malignancy).
- Refeeding syndrome.

- Effect of nutrition on disease processes, tissue viability, recovery from illness and surgery.
- Legal and ethical aspects of withholding and withdrawing life-sustaining treatments.
- Epidemiology of nutrition and malnutrition.
- How to calculate the body mass index (BMI).
- Most appropriate feeding route and knowledge of when to refer to other specialists/departments.
- Wernicke's encephalopathy.

Questions

Question 202

A 94-year-old man confided in the geriatrician that he had found it hard to cook and to maintain a healthy diet. He said he felt tired all the time and also quite irritable. On examination, he had red spots on his shins. His hair appeared to fracture easily, coil like a corkscrew or bend in several places, leading to a 'swan-neck deformity'. What is a reasonable first step in management?

A. blood test for vitamin C

B. niacin replacement

C. riboflavin replacement

D. thiamine replacement

E. vitamin C supplementation

Question 203

A 92-year-old complains of marked lethargy, has unintentionally lost 20% of her body weight in the past four months and has had very little nutritional intake for 15 days. She has a history of alcohol misuse and has been self-administering antacids to help with symptoms of heart burn. Admission bloods show electrolyte and fluid imbalance, and ketones are found in her urine. How should recommencement of nutrition be implemented?

A. correction of electrolyte and fluid imbalances before feeding is not necessary

B. oral thiamine 100 mg once a day

C. starting nutrition support at a maximum of 10 kcal/kg/day, increasing levels slowly to meet or exceed full needs by day 4–7

D. starting nutrition support at a maximum of 20 kcal/kg/day, increasing levels slowly to meet or exceed full needs by day 4–7

E. starting nutrition support at a maximum of 30 kcal/kg/day, increasing levels slowly to meet or exceed full needs by day 4–7

Question 204

You are asked by nursing staff to review the position of a nasogastric (NG) feeding tube so that feeding of a 68-year-old man, who has suffered a haemorrhagic stroke, can commence. He has a past medical history of chronic obstructive pulmonary disease and takes a number of medications to control his symptoms. The NG tube was flushed with water before insertion, and the X-ray shows a hyperexpanded chest and the tube line deviating out to the left from around mid-thorax distally (level of T5). The pH of aspirated fluid is measured at 4.9. Which of the following is the most appropriate intervention?

A. begin feeding and watch for any symptoms of coughing

B. leave the tube overnight, flush the tube with water and recheck the position the following day

C. remove the nasogastric tube

D. repeat the chest X-ray to recheck the position

E. repeat the pH testing

Question 205

A 72-year-old man with a history of alcohol abuse is brought to the emergency department by the police, who found him lying down by the side of the street. On examination, he is somnolent and confused. He has a horizontal gaze palsy with impaired vestibulo-ocular reflexes and severe truncal ataxia in the presence of normal motor strength and muscle stretch reflexes. MRI brain was normal. What is the appropriate immediate management?

A. carbohydrate only

B. multivitamin only

C. thiamine: 100–200 mg orally once daily; 100 mg intramuscularly once daily

D. thiamine: 250–500 mg intravenously every eight hours, magnesium sulphate: 2–4 g/day intravenously and multivitamin supplements

E. thiamine: 250–500 mg intravenously every eight hours, and multivitamin supplements

Question 206

The daughter of one of the patients on your ward is concerned about their parent's nutritional state. She asks you whether nutritional support would be helpful. Which of the following scenarios would meet the definition criteria for malnutrition?

A. body mass index less than 20 kg/m^2
B. diagnosis of inflammatory bowel disease
C. small oral intake for the last five days
D. unintentional weight loss greater than 5% over the last three months
E. unintentional weight loss greater than 10% over the last six months

Question 207

An 80-year-old presents with weight loss. On further questioning he reports pain on eating food, which he had put down to his angina. He denies dysphagia, abdominal pain, vomiting, changes in bowel habit or jaundice. His past medical history includes gastro-oesophageal reflux disease, hypercholesterolaemia, hypertension, ischaemic heart disease, osteoporosis, fracture left hip in 2018 and type 2 diabetes. Current drug history includes a calcium and vitamin D supplement, aspirin 75 mg od, alendronate 70 mg once a week, amlodipine 5 mg od, GTN spray as required, nicorandil 30 mg bd and omeprazole 20 mg od. On examination, he has a BMI of 18 kg/m^2. There are no cardiac murmurs, chest is clear, abdomen is soft and non-tender with no organomegaly. On examination of the mouth, you find dentures and a deep punched ulcer at the right buccal mucosa. You arrange a biopsy which does not show any malignant changes. What is the most likely cause of the ulceration?

A. alendronate
B. aspirin
C. Crohn's disease
D. nicorandil
E. ulcerative colitis

Answers for Chapter 10

202 Correct Answer: E

Explanation: The diagnosis of scurvy is primarily a clinical one, based on a dietary history of inadequate vitamin C intake and the various manifestations described above. The combination of follicular hyperkeratosis and perifollicular haemorrhage is pathognomonic and occurs early in the disease. Vitamin C needs replacing, not the other vitamins. Subjective improvement commonly begins within 24 hours, and the lethargy, anorexia and pain diminish in two to three days. Joint swelling resolves in a few days. The purplish hue of the skin lesions pales quickly and then subsides in two to four weeks, leaving areas of brown pigmentation that slowly disappear.

Reading

Hirschmann JV, Raugi GJ. Adult scurvy. *J Am Acad Dermatol* 1999; 41 (6): 895–910. www.nhs.uk/conditions/scurvy/.

203 Correct Answer: C

Explanation: She is at high risk of the 'refeeding' syndrome'. The prescription for people at high risk of developing refeeding problems should consider:

- Starting nutrition support at a maximum of 10 kcal/kg/day, increasing levels slowly to meet or exceed full needs by four to seven days.
- Using only 5 kcal/kg/day in extreme cases (for example, BMI less than 14 kg/m^2 or negligible intake for more

than 15 days) and monitoring cardiac rhythm continually in these people and any others who already have or develop any cardiac arrhythmias.

- Restoring circulatory volume and monitoring fluid balance and overall clinical status closely.

- Providing immediately before and during the first ten days of feeding: oral thiamine 200–300 mg daily, vitamin B co strong one or two tablets three times a day (or full dose daily intravenous vitamin B preparation, if necessary) and a balanced multivitamin/trace element supplement once daily.

- Providing oral, enteral or intravenous supplements of potassium (likely requirement 2–4 mmol/kg/day), phosphate (likely requirement 0.3–0.6 mmol/kg/day) and magnesium (likely requirement 0.2 mmol/kg/day intravenous, 0.4 mmol/kg/day oral) unless pre-feeding plasma levels are high. Pre-feeding correction of low plasma levels is unnecessary.

Reading

www.nice.org.uk/guidance/cg32/chapter/1-guidance.

204 Correct Answer: C

Explanation: Although the National Patient Safety Agency says that nasogastric feeding tubes are safe to use when the pH of aspirate is between 1 and 5.5, it specifically counsels not to flush tubes with water before use. This is because a falsely reassuring pH can be obtained due to mixing of water and tube lubricant. This fits with the clinical picture here where the tube is deviating at the level of the carina and is directed down into the left lung. Due to hyper-expansion of the lung because of emphysema, often the end of the tube can appear below the diaphragm, when, in fact, it is not.

Feeding is likely to introduce fluid directly into the lung and result in aspiration pneumonia. Although the pH suggests the tube is in the right place, the CXR positioning is clearly abnormal, and there is no value therefore in repeating the CXR in this case. When looking at the X-ray, the nasogastric tube should remain in the midline down to the level of the diaphragm. Flushing the tube with water first makes pH testing invalid. Hence any repeat testing may also be falsely reassuring with respect to tube position. Because the position is recognised to be abnormal on the X-ray and NPSA guidance is clear that tubes should not be flushed before testing, removal and reinsertion are essential.

205 Correct Answer: D

Explanation: The scenario describes a presentation with Wernicke's encephalopathy. Operational criteria have been proposed to guide the presumptive diagnosis by requiring two out of the four conditions:

- Dietary deficiency.
- Oculomotor abnormalities.
- Cerebellar dysfunction.
- Altered mental state or mild memory impairment.

The majority of patients who present with this condition have a degree of altered level of consciousness or cognitive dysfunction. It can vary from mild irritability, mental slowing, impaired concentration and apathy to frank confusion, delirium, coma and death. Patients may also present with various psychiatric manifestations, including acute psychosis. A history of alcohol dependence, poor dietary intake, vomiting, diarrhoea, fever, co-existing conditions, immunodeficiency or recent abdominal surgery should be elicited. The sensitivity of both CT and MRI are low, so these are not reliable in ruling out the diagnosis. These patients must be stabilised. Airway protection by appropriate means is necessary depending on the level of consciousness, and intravenous access should be promptly established. Thiamine should be administered before carbohydrate administration. A low dose may be insufficient given the poor blood-brain barrier permeability of thiamine. It is important to correct any magnesium deficiency simultaneously (monitor and correct magnesium levels appropriately) and supplement with other water-soluble vitamins (such as nicotinamide and pyridoxine), because persons at risk for thiamine deficiency are commonly at risk.

Reading

Thomson AD, Marshall EJ. BNF Recommendations for the treatment of Wernicke's encephalopathy: Lost in translation? *Alcohol and Alcoholism* 2013; 48: 514–515.

206 Correct Answer: E

Explanation: Malnutrition is an indication for nutritional support and is defined by any of the following scenarios:

- Body mass index (BMI) of less than 18.5 kg/m^2.
- Unintentional weight loss >10% within the last three to six months.

- BMI of less than 20 kg/m^2 and unintentional weight loss >5% within the last three to six months.

'At risk' of malnutrition is defined as any of:

- Poor food intake for more than five days and/or are likely to eat little or nothing for five days or longer.
- Poor absorptive capacity and/or high nutrient losses and/or increased nutritional needs from causes such as catabolism.

Reading

National Institute for Health and Care Excellence. Nutrition support for adults: Oral nutrition support, enteral tube feeding and parenteral nutrition. Clinical Guideline [CG32]. www.nice.org.uk/ guidance/cg32.

207 Correct Answer: D

Explanation: This patient has a deep, painful oral ulcer without any features suggestive of inflammatory bowel disease. Nicorandil is the most likely drug to cause this type of oral ulceration. Nicorandil is a drug used second line in the prophylaxis and treatment of stable angina. Ulceration occurs in 0.4% to 5% of people taking nicorandil, usually occurring one to 36 months from initiation of treatment. Alendronate and aspirin can cause gastro-oesophageal ulceration.

Reading

McGettigan P, Ferner RE. Painful perianal ulcers with nicorandil. *BMJ* 15 September 2020; 370: m3351.

11

Rehabilitation and Transfers of Care

LEARNING OBJECTIVE:

A key aim of this part of the curriculum is to have the knowledge and skills to provide rehabilitation to an older person in a variety of acute and community settings and be able to confidently manage frail people in a hospital-at-home, intermediate care and community setting (home or care home) and to provide a community geriatric medicine service.

Rehabilitation

Areas to cover are:

- The 'rehabilitation ethos' and principles of rehabilitation (including goal setting, use of assessment scales).
- Goal setting in rehabilitation and use of assessment scales.
- Evidence base for rehabilitation.
- Assessment of patients for rehabilitation in medical, orthopaedic and surgical wards.
- Prevalence of frailty in different settings: community, care homes, acute admissions and inpatients.
- Physical therapies to improve muscle strength and function.
- Adverse outcomes of frailty in different settings: community and inpatients.
- Evidence-based interventions to improve outcomes for frail older people in a range of settings.
- Therapeutic techniques/training to improve balance and gait.
- Aids and appliances which reduce disability.
- Specialist rehabilitation services (including orthogeriatric and stroke).
- The impact of cognitive impairment on rehabilitation.
- General awareness of the financial support available to patients and their carers.
- Assessment methods/processes undertaken to access services (including the unified single assessment process).
- Rôle and referral to independent mental capacity advocates (IMCAs).
- Structure, rôle and responsibilities of the multidisciplinary team, including the importance of outside agencies, and the way in which individual behaviours can impact on a group.
- Selection of patients for rehabilitation.
- Managing acute illness safely in community settings, including hospital-at-home services.
- Principles of community-based rehabilitation.

Transfers of Care and Discharge

Areas to cover are:

- Appropriate discharge plan and anticipatory care planning.
- Resources available following discharge, e.g. intermediate care, community care, domiciliary care, voluntary sector support, respite care, institution-based long-term care, health service–funded long-term care.
- Rôle of the geriatrician and the multidisciplinary team in discharge planning in the liaison with GPs, carers and specialty community services (e.g. heart failure, COPD), with an understanding of the structure, rôle and responsibilities of the multidisciplinary team (including the importance of outside agencies and the way in which individual behaviours can impact on a group).
- Importance of prompt and accurate information sharing with primary care.
- Awareness of the financial support available to patients and their carers.
- Medical involvement in all discharge planning, including where patients wish to self-charge.

Questions

Question 208

A 79-year-old man is currently on your rehabilitation ward following a fall and subsequent surgery for a fractured neck of femur. Prior to admission, he mobilised with a single walking stick but has now been advised to use a walking frame. He asks you about the rationale for the change of walking aid and how he should safely use it. Which of the following statements is correct?

A. frames can be used to help with standing up from a sitting position

B. frames enable a greater proportion of body weight to be offloaded from the legs compared to walking sticks

C. frames increase stability when walking on wet floors

D. frames promote a forward-leaning posture

E. lightweight frames should be carried up and down stairs

Question 209

An 81-year-old woman usually lives alone in a bungalow. She is currently recovering in hospital following pneumonia. Her past medical history includes ischaemic heart disease and Parkinson's disease. Despite optimal medical management, her balance has deteriorated. Prior to admission, she was able to walk around her property without any aids. The multidisciplinary team now feel she needs something to help her balance and lower her risk of falling around her home. She wishes to be able to carry things, such as meals and hot drinks, from her kitchen to her living room at times when nobody else is in her property. Her home has quite wide doorways but contains a number of turns to navigate. Which of the following walking aids would be most suitable for her needs?

A. a four-wheeled household trolley

B. a four-wheeled walking frame with an attached tray

C. a non-wheeled walking frame with an attached tray

D. a single walking stick

E. a two-wheeled walking frame with an attached tray

Question 210

Which of the following statements regarding walking sticks is correct?

A. correct length is the handle at level of wrist crease with arms hanging freely at sides while standing bare-footed

B. people with dementia benefit equally to people without dementia

C. sticks with crook handles tend to be less comfortable to use

D. tripod sticks aid weight transfer when climbing flights of stairs

E. white sticks with red stripes indicate that the user has complete visual loss

Question 211

Which duration of moderate-intensity exercise is recommended as the minimum each week for people over the age of 65 living in the UK?

A. 60 minutes

B. 75 minutes

C. 120 minutes

D. 150 minutes

E. 180 minutes

Question 212

Based on currently available evidence, which of the following interventions is most likely to improve the physical function of older people with frailty in acute care settings?

A. comprehensive geriatric assessment

B. medication review

C. nutritional support intervention

D. physical exercise intervention

E. vitamin D supplementation

Question 213

Which of the following beneficial effects is most likely to be realised by performing discharge planning?

A. financial cost savings

B. improved patient independence

C. reduced 90-day readmission rates

D. reduced healthcare-associated infection rates

E. reduced in-hospital mortality

Question 214

According to the King's Fund, which of the following is the most accurate description of the term 'rehabilitation'?

A. a holistic assessment that guides multidisciplinary intervention for chronic disease

B. a process aiming to restore personal autonomy in those aspects of daily living considered most relevant by patients or service users and their family carers

C. a process of assisting people with disabilities in improving, recovering or limiting decline

D. a process to enable people to fulfil, or to work towards fulfilling, their potential as occupational beings

E. a process to restore daily living skills in older people recovering from acute illness

Question 215

Which of the following statements is most true about 'goal setting' in geriatric rehabilitation?

A. adult rehabilitation and geriatric rehabilitation follow identical goal-setting processes

B. goal setting is independent of level of communication skills

C. in clinical trials, 'care as usual' is always assumed to involve no goal setting

D. goal setting also includes negotiation of goals

E. patients who are frail never need guidance in defining their rehabilitation goals

Question 216

Which of the following is said to encourage independence and enhance health in care homes?

A. a lack of financial and clinical accountability for the health of the defined population

B. a narrow focus on medical rather than holistic needs

C. few system-wide incentives around preventative care across health and social care providers

D. reducing, delaying or preventing the need for formal social care service

E. variations in policy, process and supporting systems (such as information technology) across organisations

Question 217

Which of the following statements regarding long-term care in European countries is true?

A. countries that put greater emphasis on state-supported informal care include the Netherlands

B. in most European countries, retirement ages and the participation of women in the workforce are increasing

C. it is still the case that the majority of residents admitted to long-term care are subsequently discharged

D. regulatory systems from residential care can be easily applied to home care

E. residents in nursing homes tend to live with single medical conditions

Question 218

Which one of the following is most characteristic of 'hospital-at-home'?

A. hospital-at-home applies to any patient discharged from hospital

B. hospital-at-home starts only when patients fulfil clinical criteria, live in a geographical area and both patient and caregiver accept home care

C. the hospital-at-home team can visit the patient three months after a hospital admission or a visit to the emergency department

D. the hospital-at-home team cares for patients for a few months typically

E. the hospital-at-home team does not need a defined geographical area

Question 219

In the context of taking a history for geriatric rehabilitation, an open question such as 'What would you like to be able to do that you cannot do now?' probes which of the following constructs?

A. anatomy

B. disability

C. handicap

D. impairment

E. pathology

Question 220

A 'good advance care planning discussion' could be characterised by which one of the following?

A. a follow-up review is usually not needed

B. an introduction of the concept is usually unnecessary

C. a single template is useful

D. discussions should be characterised by truthfulness, respect, time, compassion and empathy

E. discussions usually need to take place on more than one occasion (over days, weeks, months) and should not be completed on a single visit in most circumstances

Question 221

Which of the following is unlikely to be included in a discharge plan?

A. advice about welfare and benefits

B. arrangements for ongoing health support

C. details about the patient's condition

D. details of useful community and voluntary organisations

E. information about medicines now being taken

Question 222

A year ago, an 82-year-old man with dementia had moved with his wife into a privately owned bungalow. He received assistance from home care services four times a day, and the occupational therapists had provided him with several aids and appliances, including a pressure-relieving mattress. However, his wife contacted the general practitioner to say that she was exhausted and stressed because he had been screaming out regularly during the night. He slept with a dim night light. She had to provide a significant amount of care for her husband, especially at night. His condition had

not recently changed. What is the most appropriate next step in management?

A. admit the husband to acute hospital via the emergency department

B. community psychiatric nurse to visit

C. domiciliary visit from a geriatrician

D. respite care for husband and apply for increased care funding

E. transfer husband to nursing home

Question 223

A carer explains why his wife needed to go to a care home: 'I needed more assistance from others and could not get it.' What scale might have been useful to probe into this?

A. ADL

B. BRS-D

C. CES-D

D. IADL

E. Instrumental support scale

Question 224

Which of the following most promotes ineffective care transitions?

A. advance care planning

B. anticipation of post-discharge needs and inadequate post-discharge care plans

C. effective transfer of critical information between health professionals for post-discharge planning, including follow-up

D. engagement with caregivers

E. failure to identify patients at risk of readmission

Question 225

A 74-year-old woman is recovering from pneumonia on your ward. Her past history includes Alzheimer's dementia that was diagnosed three years ago. Despite this, prior to admission she lived alone and was mainly independent, only relying on her daughter's assistance for shopping and handling her finances. She has now completed her course of antibiotics but can only mobilise short distances with the assistance of two staff members and a wheeled walking frame. Which of the following statements is correct regarding rehabilitation for people with dementia?

A. implicit teaching methods are more effective than explicit ones

B. including carers in rehabilitation sessions reduces efficacy via distraction

C. physical activity will increase falls risk and should be minimised

D. rehabilitation is ineffective for people with moderate to severe dementia

E. repetition of tasks should be avoided to prevent frustration

Question 226

Which of the outcomes is most likely for an older person with physical frailty undergoing a 12-week supervised programme of resistance training?

A. 10% increase in leg muscle strength

B. 20% increase in muscle mass

C. 30% improvement in gait speed

D. higher risk of injury

E. no change in falls risk

Question 227

The use of hospital-at-home services to prevent hospital admissions for older people is associated with the greatest benefit in which of the following criteria?

A. carer satisfaction

B. financial cost

C. probability of living in a care home at six months

D. six-month mortality rate

E. subsequent hospital admission rates when compared to readmissions among those initially admitted to hospital

Question 228

An 86-year-old woman is currently an inpatient on the stroke rehabilitation unit. She has an in-dwelling urinary catheter, which has been placed to protect her skin from damage related to urinary incontinence. She has a grade 2 pressure ulcer on her sacrum. Staff notice her urine is cloudy and send a sample for urine culture. The patient is clinically well and apyrexial.

Which action is most appropriate?

TABLE 11.1

Investigations.

Urine culture	Significant growth of *E. coli*. sensitive to trimethoprim

A. commence course of trimethoprim

B. observe

C. remove urinary catheter

D. repeat the urine culture

E. replace urinary catheter

Answers for Chapter 11

208 Correct Answer: B

Explanation: Walking frames allow a greater degree of weight to be offloaded from the legs compared to walking sticks (estimated up to two thirds of weight compared to one quarter). All walking aids can potentially improve balance and can help adopt a more upright posture. Walking aids do not improve stability on wet floors. In damp situations like bathrooms, fixed grab rails would be a safer option. Frames should not be used to aid standing upright. The arms of chairs should support body weight when standing, with the frame only being held once up on one's feet. Frames should not be carried on the stairs. When required, separate frames should be provided for upstairs and downstairs use.

Reading

Disability Living Foundation. Choosing walking equipment. www.dlf.org.uk/pdfs/choosing_walking_equipment.pdf.

209 Correct Answer: B

Explanation: A walking stick would enable one hand to be free to potentially carry other objects, but this would be likely to impair her balance. In addition, people with Parkinson's disease can find using walking sticks difficult due to loss of arm swing and the stop-start nature of the movement (this is also true for non-wheeled frames). A non-wheeled frame needs to be lifted up between steps. A two-wheeled walker can be pushed along in straight lines but is likely to need to be lifted to turn around corners. So, these two options probably won't help her carry objects around. A four-wheeled household trolley is not a mobility aid and should not be used to improve gait stability. A four-wheeled walker is likely to be the best option, although clearly not without risk, in this clinical scenario. Typically, the front wheels pivot to allow movement around corners without lifting, it would aid fluidity of movement for someone with Parkinson's disease and it can be fitted with a tray for carrying objects. The use of four-wheeled walkers may be limited by available space indoors. Wheeled walkers tend to be better for improving balance rather than offloading weight due to the tendency to roll forwards.

Reading

Disability Living Foundation. Choosing walking equipment. www.dlf.org.uk/pdfs/choosing_walking_equipment.pdf.

210 Correct Answer: C

Explanation: To establish the correct length of a walking stick or frame, the patient should stand in usual footwear with arms freely hanging by sides (natural 15-degree flex), and the handle should be at level of wrist crease. People with moderate to severe dementia can have difficulty learning how to use walking aids correctly and can forget to use them when mobilising. Sticks with crook handles (curved) can be looped over the arm when not being used but tend to be less comfortable to use than other designs. Right-angle handles help transfer more weight through the stick. Anatomically moulded (Fischer) sticks come in left- and right-handed versions. They help to spread weight more evenly and can help people with painful hand conditions such as arthritis. Tripod or quadrupod sticks are bulkier. They improve stability on flat surfaces but are not to be used on stairs or uneven surfaces. White sticks indicate blindness. The addition of red stripes is for combined deafness and blindness.

211 Correct Answer: D

Explanation: Adults aged 65 and over should aim to be physically active every day and do activities that improve strength, balance and flexibility on at least two days a week. A minimum of 150 minutes of moderate intensity activity a week or 75 minutes of vigorous intensity activity (or a combination of both) is recommended. They are also advised to reduce time spent sitting or lying down and break up long periods of not moving with some activity. Exercises to improve strength, balance and flexibility are advised for those who have fallen or feel at risk of falling. Moderate intensity activities include brisk walking/hiking, slow cycling, dancing, pushing a lawn mower and doubles tennis.

Reading

www.nhs.uk/live-well/exercise/physical-activity-guidelines-older-adults/.

212 Correct Answer: A

Explanation: Very little evidence currently exists for the benefit of interventions to improve outcomes of people with frailty in acute care settings. The best evidence base is for CGA for people both with and without frailty.

Reading

Dent E, Martin FC, Bergman H, et al. Management of frailty: Opportunities, challenges, and future directions. *Lancet* 2019; 394: 1376–1386.

213 Correct Answer: C

Explanation: Discharge planning probably results in a small reduction in hospital length of stay and reduces the risk of readmission to hospital at three months follow-up for older people with a medical condition. It may also increase satisfaction for patients and healthcare professionals. There is little evidence that discharge planning reduces financial costs or improves other metrics.

Reading

Gonçalves-Bradley DC, Lannin NA, Clemson LM, et al. Discharge planning from hospital. *Cochrane Database Syst Rev* 2016; (1). Art. No.: CD000313.

214 Correct Answer: B

Explanation: Rehabilitation carries the basic aim of assisting people with disabilities in improving, recovering or limiting decline in physical, mental and social skills. The King's Fund defines rehabilitation as 'a process aiming to restore personal autonomy in those aspects of daily living considered most relevant by patients or service users and their family carers'. The definition of occupational therapy is a process to enable people to fulfil, or to work towards fulfilling, their potential as occupational beings (option C). The others are all true but are not the King's Fund definition of 'rehabilitation'.

Reading

Stott JD, Quinn TJ. Principles of rehabilitation of older people. *Medicine* 2017; 45: 1–5.

215 Correct Answer: D

Explanation: Goal setting is regarded as an essential part of rehabilitation. It has been defined as the establishment or negotiation of rehabilitation goals and refers to the intended future state of the patient, which will usually involve a change from the current situation.

Reading

Smit EB, Bouwstra H, Hertogh CM, et al. Goal-setting in geriatric rehabilitation: A systematic review and meta-analysis. *Clin Rehabil* 2019; 33 (3): 395–407.

216 Correct Answer: D

Explanation: People maintain their independence as far as possible by reducing, delaying or preventing the need for formal social care services. The care for people who are living in care homes or who are at risk of losing their independence is being held back by a series of care barriers, financial barriers and organisational barriers.

Reading

The framework for enhanced health in care homes. NHS England, March 2020. www.england.nhs.uk/wp-content/uploads/2020/03/the-framework-for-enhanced-health-in-care-homes-v2-0.pdf.

217 Correct Answer: B

Explanation: In most European countries, retirement ages and the participation of women in the workforce are increasing. Rising long-term care (LTC) expenditure will be a problem both for countries with high reliance on formal care, such as the Netherlands, and for those which provide greater emphasis on state-supported informal care, such as the United Kingdom. It is still the case that the majority of residents admitted to LTC are not subsequently discharged. Residents in nursing homes have polypharmacy and multimorbidity, and these are particularly difficult to manage when coupled to the prognostic uncertainty already described. A challenge to increased reliance on informal care is quality assurance. The regulatory systems for LTC facilities would be both inappropriate and impractical in the context of care delivered between a husband and wife or between generations of the same family.

Reading

Jos M. G. A. Schols and Adam Gordon. Chapter 37, Long-term care: Residential and nursing home care: From the past to the future. In *Oxford textbook of geriatric medicine* (Third edition). Eds. Jean-Pierre Michel, B. Lynn Beattie, Finbarr C. Martin, Jeremy Walston, 2017. Oxford: Oxford University Press. DOI: 10.1093/med/9780198701590.001.0001.

218 Correct Answer: B

Explanation: Features of 'hospital-at-home':

- The hospital-at-home team is composed of doctors and nurses.
- Identification of a specific group of suitable candidates.
- Defined geographical area.
- Hospital-at-home starts only when patients fulfil clinical criteria, live in a geographical area and both patient and caregiver accept home care.
- Hospital-at-home team can visit the patient daily.
- Hospital-at-home team can visit the patient on the day of discharge after hospital admission or a visit to the emergency department.
- Hospital-at-home team cares for patients for a short period of time (generally not more than 10–15 days).
- A report at the end of care.
- Hospital-at-home outcomes should be analogous to conventional admission care.

Reading

Escarrabill J. Discharge planning and home care for end-stage COPD patients. *Eur Respir J* 2009; 34 (2): 507–512.

219 Correct Answer: C

Explanation: This is a question probing the definition 'handicap'.

Important definitions include:

Pathology: abnormality of structure or function affecting an organ or organ system—for example, osteoarthritis, ischaemic heart disease.

Impairment: any loss or abnormality of psychological, physiological or anatomical structure or function—for example, joint pain, breathlessness, muscle weakness, visual impairment, deafness.

Disability: any restriction or lack of ability to perform a task or activity—for example, walking, dressing, going up and down stairs, hearing.

Handicap: the disadvantages for a particular individual resulting from an impairment or disability that limits or prevents fulfilment of a rôle which is normal for someone of that age, sex or culture—for example, reading a newspaper, going to shops or the pub, gardening, attending a football match, playing the piano.

This question is not a test of anatomy, in the context of a rehabilitation assessment.

Reading

Young J, Robinson J, Dickinson E. Rehabilitation for older people. *BMJ* 1998; 316 (7138): 1108–1109.

220 Correct Answer: D

Explanation: The individual needs to be ready for the discussion—it cannot be forced. Discussions usually need to take place on more than one occasion (over days, weeks, months) and should not be completed on a single visit in most circumstances. Discussions take time and effort and cannot be completed as a simple checklist exercise. Discussions should take place in comfortable, unhurried surroundings; time is a key factor. A step-by-step approach should be used. It is important that capacity is maximised by ensuring the treatment of any transient condition affecting communication and optimising sensory function (e.g. by obtaining the patient's hearing aid). Discussions should be characterised by truthfulness, respect, time, compassion and empathy. A tool to introduce the concept and guide the discussion may help professionals to address advance care planning with patients.

Reading

National guidelines, 2009 RCP/BGS/NCPC/BSRM/ Alzheimer's Society. Concise guidance to good practice. A series of evidence-based guidelines for clinical management. No. 12: Advance care planning.   www.bgs.org.uk/sites/default/files/content/ attachment/2018-04-18/Advance%20Care%20 Planning%20Guideline.pdf/.

221 Correct Answer: A

Explanation: Staff should produce a discharge plan, give a copy to the patient and forward one promptly to the patient's GP and care home if that is the destination of discharge.

A discharge plan includes information such as:

• Details about your condition.
• Information about medicines you are now taking.
• Contact information after discharge, including who to contact and how to contact them with any questions about your care.
• Arrangements for continuing social care support, aids and equipment.
• Arrangements for ongoing health support.
• Details of useful community and voluntary organisations.

Reading

Age UK. Factsheet 37. Hospital discharge. August 2019. www.ageuk.org.uk/globalassets/age-uk/documents/ factsheets/fs37_hospital_discharge_fcs.pdf.

222 Correct Answer: D

Explanation: There is no medical or physical health reason to admit him to hospital or require a geriatrician domiciliary visit or district nurse. He has a relatively good care package and adaptations in place, but carer burden is the main issue here. Respite would be a preferred option in this scenario to provide carer relief in an attempt to avoid placement into a care home.

223 Correct Answer: E

Explanation: The instrumental support scale probes into carer subjective support. It is a 'scale', with a single item concerning the carers' perceived need for more help, a scale measuring the tasks and time provided by others and whether others help care for the patient.

Other scales referred to in this question are:

* Patient behaviour—BRS-D.
* ADL, IADL, Rosow-Breslau scales relate to physical functioning.
* CES-D (caregiver emotional health) is a single question measuring life satisfaction and multi-item scale measuring stress symptoms.

Reading

Buhr GT, Kuchibhatla M, Clipp EC. Caregivers' reasons for nursing home placement: Clues for improving discussions with families prior to the transition. *Gerontologist* February 2006; 46 (1): 52–61.

224 Correct Answer: E

Explanation: Common problems that cause ineffective care transitions:

* Failure to identify patients at risk of readmission.
* Failure to anticipate post-discharge needs and inadequate post-discharge care plans.
* Inadequate hand-over of critical information between health professionals for post-discharge planning, including follow-up.
* Failure to identify individuals who may be involved in the patient's

caregiving who need to be educated about the post-discharge care plan.

* Failure to engage and educate patients and caregivers.
* Poor social or financial resources with inadequate access to nutrition and transportation.
* Poor health literacy and failure to understand discharge plans.
* Polypharmacy and poor medication management.
* Failure to adequately address advance care planning.

Reading

Elizabeth C. Gundersen, Benjamin A. Bensadon, and Joseph G. Ouslandern. Chapter 39, Transitions between care settings until death. In *Oxford textbook of geriatric medicine* (Third edition). Eds. Jean-Pierre Michel, B. Lynn Beattie, Finbarr C. Martin, Jeremy Walston. Oxford: Oxford University Press, 2017. DOI: 10.1093/med/9780198701590.001.0001.

225 Correct Answer: A

Explanation: People should not be excluded from rehabilitation simply due to a diagnosis of dementia. Promoting mobility has physical, mood and cognitive benefits. Implicit (e.g. task-based) teaching methods are usually more effective than explicit (e.g. verbal instruction) ones. Procedural learning (e.g. practice of tasks) is effective for skills known previously. Learning new techniques is challenging for people with dementia. Repetition of tasks is required. Carers can positively assist with rehabilitation. Dementia affects people differently, and an individualised approach will be required to find the most effective method of rehabilitation.

Reading

McGough E, Kirk Sanchez N. Rehabilitation in dementia. In *A comprehensive guide to rehabilitation of the older patient*. Ed. O'Hanlon S, Smith M., 2020.

226 Correct Answer: A

Explanation: Resistance training alone or combined with other training types (e.g. gait and balance) is associated with improvements in muscle mass and strength and reductions in falls and functional impairment. Not all studies, however, have found improvements in all of these areas. After 12 weeks, reported benefits include muscle mass increase (3%–8%), gait speed increase (6%–19%) and leg muscle strength improvement (7%–37%).

Reading

Lopez P, Pinto RS, Radaelli R, et al. Benefits of resistance training in physically frail elderly: A systematic review. *Aging Clin Exp Res* 2018; 30: 889–899.

227 Correct Answer: C

Explanation: A systematic review found that admission avoidance hospital-at-home probably makes little or no difference to six-monthly mortality and hospital transfers (compared to readmissions). It may be beneficial for patient satisfaction, but there is little data on carer satisfaction. Financial costs may be lower, but only if the costs of informal care provision are excluded. There is some evidence (although rated as low-certainty) that the six-month probability of residing in a care home is reduced.

Reading

Shepperd S, Iliffe S, Doll HA, et al. Admission avoidance hospital-at-home. *Cochrane Database Syst Rev* 2016; (9). Art. No.: CD007491.

228 Correct Answer: C

Explanation: Urine culture should only be requested when signs of infection are present (e.g. rigors, fever, delirium, sepsis, etc.), not because the appearance or smell of the urine could suggest infection. In this case, the urine culture should not have been requested in the first instance, so no action is required other than to observe the patient. The urine culture result is likely to represent asymptomatic bacteriuria, and antibiotic treatment is not indicated in the absence of signs of infection. Indeed, inappropriate use of antibiotics may lead to antibiotic-resistant strains (making future infections more difficult to manage) and can increase the risk of *Clostridium difficile*. Replacing the urinary catheter requires further instrumentation of the urinary tract and is not without its risks. Also, there is no evidence that replacing a urinary catheter provides benefit in asymptomatic bacteriuria. The urinary catheter should be removed at the earliest opportunity when clinically appropriate. However, the scenario suggests an ongoing benefit from the catheter to protect her damaged skin. Removing the catheter based purely on the urine culture result is inappropriate.

Reading

SIGN guidelines on suspected bacterial urinary tract infection in adults. www.sign.ac.uk/media/1051/sign88.pdf.

12

Specialty Topics

Palliative Care

LEARNING OBJECTIVE:

To have the knowledge and skills required to assess and manage patients with life-limiting diseases (malignant and non-malignant) across all healthcare settings, in conjunction with other healthcare professionals.

Areas to cover are:

- Rôle of palliative care team and other agencies.
- Assessment of physical and mental state.
- Awareness of palliative care in various geriatric settings (cancer, heart failure, COPD, renal failure, stroke, dementia, Parkinson's disease, severe frailty).
- Pharmacological and non-pharmacological management of common symptoms in life-limiting illnesses such as end-stage dementia, heart failure, COPD (including pain, nausea, vomiting, constipation, breathlessness, excess respiratory tract secretions, anxiety, agitation).
- Pathophysiology of pain, including types of pain—nociceptive, visceral, neuropathic and incident.
- Polypharmacy and deprescribing.
- Range of therapeutic options available for common symptoms, i.e. disease and symptom modifying treatments (palliative surgery, radiotherapy, chemotherapy, immunotherapy, hormone therapy, drugs, physical therapies, psychological interventions).
- Knowledge of commonly used medications for pain, including range of drugs and routes of administration, adjustment of dosage in frail older people, adjustment of dosage in altered metabolism, disease progression and last few days of life, problems of polypharmacy.
- Assessment and management of acute and chronic pain.
- Emergencies in palliative care, e.g. hypercalcaemia, haemorrhage, spinal cord compression, breathlessness.
- Development of a holistic advance care planning (including multidisciplinary assessment, discussion and recording).
- Assessment of prognosis (including recognising when a patient is not imminently dying but has limited physiological reserve and is at risk of sudden acute deterioration).
- The management of movement disorders from diagnosis with a shifting emphasis towards a palliative approach with disease progression.

- Current national publications regarding end-of-life care and cardiopulmonary resuscitation decisions.
- End-of-life care, including advance care planning (including support of patients/staff/relatives/carers through advance care planning—'what if' scenarios).
- Recognition of the dying phase of terminal illness.
- Symptom profiles in terminally ill and an understanding of their pathophysiology.
- Discussion of dying, grief, abnormal grief and modern bereavement care.
- Provision of palliative care in intermediate and long-term care through liaising with other relevant agencies.

Questions

Question 229

A 63-year-old woman being treated with chemotherapy for a leukaemia is admitted to the hospital for fevers after a fall while trying to stand up from an old chair. She had diarrhoea and vomiting for two days and hasn't been eating or drinking well. She received 1.5 L intravenous saline by the paramedic team. She has had abdominal pain for two days. She has been unable to take oral medications due to nausea. No suspicious lesions are found on examination. Her airway is clear and self-maintaining. RR 24, SpO_2 100% on O_2, pulse 110, BP 86/51, GCS E4 V5 M6, pupils equal, and temperature 38.2°C. The neutrophil count is <500/mm^3. The patient is stabilised according to the ABCDE. What is the most important next management step?

A. GM-CSF

B. intravenous aminoglycoside

C. intravenous beta lactam monotherapy with piperacillin with tazobactam

D. oral antibiotics

E. prophylactic antivirals and antifungals

Question 230

Which of the following statements is most correct about deprescribing in an end-of-life context?

A. deprescribing is a relatively new concept

B. it is relatively easy to implement 'patient-based approaches' to deprescribing

C. prescriber behaviours rarely affect deprescribing

D. prescribing medicines of questionable benefit is infrequent in nursing homes

E. prescriptions of preventative drugs tend to increase on admission to a nursing home

Question 231

An 82-year-old man who has end-stage chronic obstructive pulmonary disease comes to the respiratory clinic for review. He is currently managed with tiotropium, a high-dose fluticasone/salmeterol inhaler, oral theophylline and home oxygen. Despite this, he is constantly short of breath. He is unable to walk more than a few yards. Examination confirms features of severe emphysema with a hyper-expanded chest, a respiratory rate of 25 breaths/minute at rest and bilateral poor air entry with wheeze. Oxygen saturation is 91% on 2 litres of oxygen. Arterial $pa(O_2)$ on two litres of oxygen is 8.9 kPa, and $pa(CO_2)$ is 7.8 kPa. Which of the following is the most appropriate next step to manage his breathlessness?

A. glycopyrronium

B. increased inspired oxygen

C. lorazepam

D. oramorph

E. reassurance

Question 232

An 82-year-old woman with breast cancer is in pain. She is prescribed 180 mg twice a day of controlled-release morphine (i.e. total daily dose of 360 mg). What dose of immediate-release morphine should be prescribed, when required, to relieve breakthrough pain?

A. 20 mg

B. 40 mg

C. 60 mg

D. 180 mg

E. 360 mg

Question 233

An 82-year-old man had been warned about the high risk of developing bone metastases from his prostate cancer. He now presents with spinal pain aggravated by straining (for example, at stool, or when coughing or sneezing). A diagnosis of metastatic spinal cord compression is suspected. What is the preferred neuroimaging modality?

A. MRI of the spine, including sagittal T1 and/or short T1 inversion recovery (STIR) sequences of the whole spine

B. myeolography

C. plain radiographs of the spine

D. routine MRI of the spine

E. serial imaging of the spine

Question 234

An 84-year-old patient experiences a shooting, stabbing feeling like an electric shock and a sensation of pins and needles. He also complains of symptoms of pain caused by a stimulus that does not normally provoke pain. He has been on treatment with vincristine. Which one of the following could be recommended as a pharmacological intervention for this pain in a hospital care setting that does not provide a specialist pain service?

A. cannabis sativa extract

B. capsaicin patch

C. duloxetine

D. lacosamide

E. lamotrigine

Question 235

An 85-year-old man on chemotherapy says he has been eating badly since his wife died. He attends clinic, reporting that his stools are hard, uncomfortable or difficult to pass and are less frequent than usual. He has a sense of incomplete evacuation after defaecation. He now has not opened his bowels for four days, and his abdomen does seem slightly tender and distended. He has marked halitosis. What would be a sensible approach for treatment of his problems?

A. docusate

B. glycerol suppositories

C. isaphagula husk

D. phosphate enemas

E. senna

Question 236

An 84-year-old man was diagnosed with lung cancer a few years ago. He now presents as an emergency with headaches and stridor. He is stabilised clinically, such that he no longer has life-threatening symptoms (e.g. associated stridor) and is fit enough for active treatment. A diagnosis of superior vena cava obstruction is made. A decision is made to perform a contrast enhanced spiral CT.

Which initial therapeutic option would be the most appropriate?

A. dexamethasone oral 8 mg once daily

B. dexamethasone oral 8 mg once daily + omeprazole 20 mg daily

C. dexamethasone oral 8 mg twice daily

D. dexamethasone oral 8 mg twice daily + omeprazole 20 mg daily

E. omeprazole 20 mg daily

Question 237

A 72-year-old man presents to the acute medical unit with fever, weight loss and night sweats. Chemotherapy is commenced. He receives a combination of rituximab, cyclophosphamide, doxorubicin, vincristine and prednisolone. One day later he becomes oliguric with a urine output of 5 mL/hour.

Other than fluid resuscitation, which treatment should be commenced immediately?

A. allopurinol

B. calcium supplements

TABLE 12.1

Investigations.

Serum sodium	142 mmol/L (137–144)
Serum potassium	5.8 mmol/L (3.5–4.9)
Serum urea	18.2 mmol/L (2.5–7.5)
Serum creatinine	273 μmol/L (60–110)
Serum corrected calcium	2.32 mmol/L (2.2–2.6)
Serum phosphate	1.8 mmol/L (0.8–1.4)
Serum actate dehydrogenase	856 IU/L (20–250 IU/L)
Serum urate	0.92 mmol/L (0.2–0.4 mmol/L)
Serum CRP	25 mg/L (<10)
CT chest/abdomen/ pelvis	Bulky widespread lymphadenopathy
Lymph node biopsy	Diffuse large B cell lymphoma

C. paracetamol

D. phosphate binders

E. rasburicase

Question 238

A 66-year-old woman is admitted with lower back pain, nausea and constipation. She has breast cancer with liver metastases and is taking tamoxifen. She is well known to the community palliative care team. On direct questioning she has had pain for several weeks, but over the past week it has worsened with radiation down the right thigh and pins and needles. She has had two falls at home.

Abdominal examination reveals a 2 cm liver edge and mild left iliac fossa tenderness. On neurological examination there is no spine tenderness, tone is normal, power is reduced to 4/5 bilaterally on knee flexion and dorsiflexion of right ankle but reflexes are intact and there is no sensory loss. Which of the following statements is true?

A. an urgent X-ray of the lumbosacral spine should be performed

B. further investigations are not appropriate as she has metastatic cancer and is receiving palliative care

C. high-dose steroids should be prescribed and an urgent MRI scan performed of her lumbar spine only

D. metastatic spinal cord compression is unlikely in the absence of a sensory level

E. she should be immobilised until a whole spine MRI has been urgently performed

Question 239

A 74-year-old woman has a diagnosis of renal cell carcinoma, now with liver and bone metastases. She is on regular morphine but has recently developed severe pain in her left upper arm, which does not completely respond to as-required doses of morphine. Her son reports that she has become increasingly agitated and confused over the past 24 hours and is experiencing visual hallucinations, yet remains in significant pain. The results of recent blood investigations are not available. Which of the following would be the most appropriate initial management?

A. add amitriptyline

B. increase her regular morphine dose

C. start an oral bisphosphonate for bone pain

D. stop the morphine

E. urgent referral to specialist palliative care team

Question 240

An 82-year-old man presents with delirium and constipation. His serum calcium is 3.0 mmol/L (reading range 2.2–2.6 mmol/L). An ECG shows sinus rhythm, rate 76 beats per minute, shortened QT interval. What is the immediate best management?

A. dialysis

B. frusemide

C. glucocorticoids

D. intravenous 0.9% saline

E. zolendronic acid

Question 241

According to the Gold Standards Framework prognostic indicator guidance, there are a number of general indicators of decline. Identify a correct indicator.

A. good response to treatments, decreasing reversibility

B. progressive weight loss (>5%) in past six months

C. repeated unplanned hospital admissions

D. serum albumin <30 g/L

E. stable level of functional activity

Question 242

Which of the following statements is correct concerning the ReSPECT process from the Resuscitation Council (UK)?

A. the outcome of the ReSPECT process usually does not involve the person's family

B. the ReSPECT process creates personalised recommendations for a person's clinical care and treatment in a future emergency in which they are unable to make or express choices

C. the ReSPECT process has to be completed before a DNACPR decision is made

D. the ReSPECT process is legally binding

E. the ReSPECT process is only available for persons reaching the end of their lives

Question 243

According to the Resuscitation Council (UK), which statement is correct regarding decisions about cardiopulmonary resuscitation (CPR)?

A. a 'do not attempt CPR' (DNACPR) decision overrides clinical judgement in circumstances not envisaged when that decision was made and recorded

B. CPR is advisable if a DNACPR decision is absent, even if the healthcare team is as certain as it can be that a person is dying as an inevitable result of underlying disease or a catastrophic health event

C. in the event of a cardiac arrest of a patient who made an advance decision to refuse CPR while having mental capacity, CPR should not be given

D. when CPR has no realistic prospect of success, there is usually no need to explain the need and basis for a DNACPR decision to a patient or to those close to a patient who lacks capacity

E. where a patient or those close to a patient disagree with a DNACPR decision, the doctor has the final say

---

Old Age Psychiatry

LEARNING OBJECTIVE:

To know how to assess and manage older patients presenting with the common psychiatric conditions and to know when to seek specialist advice.

Areas to cover are:

- Diagnosis of older people with psychiatric conditions (especially depression, anxiety and delusional states).
- Clinical pharmacology, therapeutics and pharmacy for older people with psychiatric conditions.
- Psychiatric assessment methods and tools (including cognitive and mood assessment).
- Overview of pharmacological and non-pharmacological interventions in psychiatric illness.
- Differentiating between cognitive impairment and other diagnoses.
- Assessment of mental capacity.
- Mental capacity and mental health legislation, and safeguarding issues/vulnerable adults.
- Ethical issues.
- Working collaboratively with other specialists, particularly old-age psychiatrists, and agencies to manage the older patient with mental ill health.

Questions

Question 244

A 76-year-old woman, with a three-year history of dementia, lives at home with her husband. She has been showing new aggressive behaviours, such as attempting to hit the paid carers during personal care, kicking, scratching, biting, spitting and 'cursing'. At night, in particular, she has been exhibiting certain non-aggressive behaviours (e.g. pacing up and down the corridor of the flat, general restlessness and repetitive mannerisms). She also appears to be experiencing disengagement with the environment around her. What would be a reasonable first step in management?

A. carbamazepine

B. haloperidol

C. non-pharmacological interventions for carers to use

D. repeated transcranial magnetic stimulation

E. tricyclic antidepressants

Question 245

Neighbours brought a 91-year-old Asian man, who lived alone in a bungalow, to the medical assessment unit of a district general hospital. The neighbours said they were concerned that he was appearing to develop dementia. Apparently, he disclosed to them experiences of witnessing people and animals in his house, including various-sized zebras and ostriches, parrots and blue fish flying across the room. He knew that these visions were not real, but he was worried about dementia being a likely diagnosis. The visions lasted for minutes to hours, and the animals were perceived to stare at him. His other medical problems included chronic asthma. He also was registered partially sighted, having been diagnosed with bilateral cataracts and macular degeneration. He had never hallucinated before. What is the likely diagnosis?

A. Anton's syndrome

B. Charles Bonnet syndrome

C. delirium

D. diffuse Lewy body disease

E. Diogenes syndrome ('senile squalor syndrome')

Question 246

A 72-year-old man appeared to remember nothing of his past, having travelled suddenly and unexpectedly to attend his ex-wife's funeral. At the funeral, he introduces himself using a different identity, and seems genuinely confused who is. He was cognitively intact otherwise. He had only sought neuropsychiatric attention once he was seeking to recover his original identity. He was a lifelong non-drinker of alcohol. What is the most likely diagnosis?

A. Alzheimer's disease

B. delirium

C. Diogenes syndrome ('senile squalor syndrome')

D. dissociative fugue

E. transient global amnesia

Question 247

An 83-year-old white woman presented with previous bilateral occipital lobe infarcts. Despite her obvious blindness, illustrated by her walking into objects, she expressed total denial of visual loss and demonstrated confabulation in her accounts of her surroundings. On examination, she demonstrated a complete loss of vision. Fundoscopy was unremarkable. Ocular movements were found to be intact if she was told in which direction to look, however she was not be able to follow a finger or light. Previous medical history included coronary artery bypass graft surgery. Which is the most likely diagnosis?

A. Anton's syndrome

B. Charles Bonnet syndrome

C. delirium

D. diffuse Lewy body disease

E. Diogenes syndrome ('senile squalor syndrome')

Question 248

A 68-year-old left-handed man presented with a three-year history of a progressive personality change. It all started with difficulty completing his work, following through on complex activities and then in maintaining his personal relationships. He also exhibited disinhibited behaviour, saying inappropriate things in public. He became dishevelled in his personal appearance and in the upkeep of his home, which was extremely disordered and cluttered from compulsive hoarding. He had amassed stacks of things in his flat, such as pornographic magazines, piles of unopened mail and other items that he had previously deemed of value such as boxes of chocolates. What is the most likely diagnosis?

A. Alzheimer's disease

B. delirium

C. Diogenes syndrome ('senile squalor syndrome')

D. dissociative fugue

E. transient global amnesia

Question 249

This question is about rating scales for depression. Which of the following is a clinician-rated ten-item scale, measuring severity of depressive symptoms; sensitive to change; mainly used to assess response to treatment but with no agreement on cut-off score for remission (between ≤4 and ≤10)?

A. Cornell scale for depression in dementia (CSDD)

B. geriatric depression scale (GDS-15)

C. hospital anxiety and depression scale (HADS)

D. Montgomery and Åsberg depression rating scale (MADRS)

E. patient health questionnaire (PHQ-9)

Question 250

Which of the following statements is true concerning alcohol use in older people?

A. diagnostic criteria and screening instruments tend to focus on past levels of alcohol intake

B. older people may be more likely than younger people to encounter the social, legal and occupational complications associated with alcohol use disorders

C. the absolute number of older people with alcohol use disorders is on the decrease

D. the presentation of older people with alcohol use disorders may be atypical (such as falls, confusion, depression) or masked by comorbid physical or psychiatric illness, which makes detection all the more difficult

E. the prevalence of alcohol use disorders in older people is generally accepted to be higher than in younger people

Question 251

An 80-year-old man is an inpatient on a department of medicine for older persons ward. A junior doctor noted multiple recent admissions, with unexplained injuries and discrepancies within the collateral history. A senior nurse on the ward highlights a strained interaction between a patient and their carer. The physiotherapist notices the patient flinching out of fear during an assessment. Finally, the dietician reflects on why a patient has such a low albumin and poor nutritional state.

What is the most likely diagnosis?

A. anorexia

B. depression

C. elder abuse

D. personality disorder

E. post-traumatic stress disorder

Question 252

An 88-year-old woman is referred with recurrent falls, deteriorating balance and increasing forgetfulness. She has been very upset recently as she has been seeing small parrots by the window. Examination showed reduced facial expression and blinking frequency, increased tone in all four limbs with hyper-reflexia but no tremor or cog-wheeling. She has a full range of eye movements, loss of red reflex but normal retinal appearance on fundoscopy. Snellen test score was 6/60 for her left eye and 3/60 for her right eye. She scored 19/30 on the Montreal Cognitive Assessment. She walked with a short-stepping gait and struggled to turn. If the visual hallucinations become distressing, what is the best management option?

A. cataract operation

B. diazepam

C. haloperidol

D. levodopa

E. quetiapine

Question 253

A 79-year-old woman with suspected Alzheimer's dementia (she had recently scored 18/30 on a Montreal Cognitive Assessment) was found by her neighbours, locked out of her house. She has a carer every morning, is not prone to wandering and usually does not leave the house without a family member. She also suffers from temporal arteritis and is on donepezil, prednisolone, calcium/vitamin D and alendronic acid. What assistive technology is she likely to benefit most from?

A. 'key safe'

B. notices reminding her to take her door key

C. pill box with alarm function

D. text message medication reminders

E. wandering monitor linked to her mobile phone

Questions

Question 254

A 92-year-old woman with vascular dementia is admitted with facial bruising and suspected head injury following a fall at home. She lived with her husband and daughter (a retired social worker with lasting power of attorney for her parents) and is dependent for all activities of daily living. Her devoted husband came in every day to help feed her. However, the ward sister observed the patient's husband slap her on the face when she refused to eat the hospital food he offered. What is the appropriate next step?

A. an independent mental capacity advocate should be consulted

B. a Protection of Older Vulnerable Adult investigation should be instigated

C. the husband's behaviour should be challenged by the ward doctor

D. the patient's daughter should be called and advised of what occurred

E. the police should be called to investigate an alleged witnessed assault

Osteoporosis and Orthogeriatrics

Osteoporosis

LEARNING OBJECTIVE:

To understand the biology and management of osteoporosis.

Areas to cover are:

- Primary and secondary causes, prevention and management of osteoporosis (drug and non-drug).
- Assessment of bone health and vitamin D deficiency/insufficiency.

- Ability to interpret bone density scans and validated assessment tools.
- The management of patients with osteoporosis with treatment failure.
- Management of patients requiring parenteral osteoporosis therapy.

Orthogeriatrics

LEARNING OBJECTIVE:

To know how to assess and manage acutely ill orthopaedic patients (including those older patients presenting with a fracture) and how to provide a comprehensive orthogeriatric and bone health service which also meets rehabilitation needs.

Areas to cover are:

- Diagnostic skills.
- Drugs and non-drug interactions.
- Planning transfers of care.
- Surgical and anaesthetic issues and understanding of postoperative care and complications (including pain control and tissue viability).
- Different models of orthogeriatric care (including rôle of intermediate care, acute trauma and orthogeriatric rehabilitation).
- Medical and surgical management of common metabolic bone diseases, e.g. osteomalacia, Paget's disease, primary hyperparathyroidism.
- Relevant national publications and guidelines including NICE and the 'Blue Book II'.
- Rôle of fracture liaison services.
- Understanding of national audits and the 'hip fracture database'.
- Maximising function through orthogeriatric rehabilitation.

Questions

Question 255

A 73-year-old man presented with a two-week history of constant low thoracic back pain after falling down half a flight of stairs. He had a past history of chronic obstructive lung disease treated with inhalers supplemented with oral prednisolone 10 mg daily; he had been unable to come off the steroids without a deterioration in his chest. On examination, there was tenderness around the low thoracic vertebrae.

TABLE 12.2

Investigations.

X-ray of the spine	T12 vertebral fracture

He is prescribed analgesia. What is the most appropriate next step?

A. contact the orthopaedic surgeon for kyphoplasty

B. reassure the patient and say that the pain will resolve spontaneously

C. request a bone density scan

D. start a bisphosphonate

E. start calcium and vitamin D supplementation

Question 256

Which one of the following is a major feature of an atypical femoral fracture, according to standardised definitions?

A. bilateral incomplete or complete femoral diaphysis fractures

B. delayed fracture healing

C. generalised increase in cortical thickness of the femoral diaphyses

D. the fracture is associated with minimal or no trauma, as in a fall from a standing height or less

E. unilateral or bilateral prodromal symptoms such as dull or aching pain in the groin or thigh

Question 257

An 82-year-old woman comes to the clinic, having suffered a left Colles' fracture after falling on ice. She smokes five cigarettes per day and has hypertension and gastro-oesophageal reflux disease. Her blood pressure is 134/84 mmHg; her pulse is 67 bpm and regular. Her body mass index (BMI) is 21 kg/m^2. She has been started on calcium and vitamin D by her general practitioner.

Which of the following is the most appropriate initial intervention?

A. continue calcium and vitamin D only

B. denosumab

C. raloxifene

D. risedronate

E. teriparatide

Question 258

Which of the following is thought to be a risk factor for osteoporosis which is independent of bone mineral density?

A. age

B. chronic liver disease

C. chronic renal disease

D. endocrine disease

E. malabsorption

Question 259

Which of the following statements is true about denosumab and its associated pathway?

A. denosumab binds with high affinity to human RANKL and blocks binding of RANKL to RANK

B. denosumab is a fully human IgG1 monoclonal antibody

C. osteonecrosis of the jaw has not been associated with denosumab

D. osteoprotegerin is a synthetic inhibitor of RANKL

E. RANK and RANKL are not expressed by endothelial cells and lymphocytes

TABLE 12.3

Investigations.

Haemoglobin	140 g/L (115–155)
White cell count	8.2 × 10⁹/L (4.0–11.0)
Platelet count	230 × 10⁹/L (150–400)
Serum sodium	141 mmol/L (135–145)
Serum potassium	4.4 mmol/L (3.5–5.0)
Serum creatinine	104 µmol/L (50–120)
Serum corrected calcium	2.4 mmol/L (2.2–2.7)
Serum albumin	45 g/L (35–55)
Serum phosphate	1.2 mmol/L (1.1–1.45)
Bone mineral density T-score	−2.8

Question 260

A 66-year-old man with epilepsy has been taking carbamazepine for 13 years, with no other significant medical history. He is on no other regular medications. He has a poor dietary intake and, although mobile, spent most of his time indoors, living a reclusive lifestyle. He was brought to the accident and emergency department following a seizure. He was cachectic, dehydrated, unkempt and unable to bear weight.

There had been no history of previous renal dysfunction.

Which is the most important contributor to his presentation?

A. acute renal failure

B. carbamazepine

C. chronic renal failure

D. primary hyperparathyroidism

E. tertiary hyperparathyroidism

Question 261

Which out of the following is the *least* common primary adverse effect of bisphosphonates?

A. acute phase response with first infusion when given intravenously

B. hypocalcaemia

C. nephrotoxicity

D. osteonecrosis of the jaw

E. upper gastrointestinal symptoms when taken orally

TABLE 12.4

Investigations.

Plasma parathyroid hormone	20.3 pmol/L (1.6–6.9)
Serum 25-hydroxyvitamin D	9 nmol/L (25–100)
Serum corrected calcium	1.87 mmol/L (2.2–2.6)
Serum creatinine	231 µmol/L (64–104)
Serum urea	25.1 mmol/L (2.5–7.8)
Serum alkaline phosphatase	467 U/L (35–120; other liver function tests normal)
Serum magnesium, phosphate and prostate-specific antigen	Normal
Myeloma screen	Normal
CT of the chest, abdomen and pelvis	Unremarkable for malignancy, however, it revealed fractures of the thoracic ribs and spine in addition to showing femoral neck fractures
X-ray	Bilateral neck of femur fractures

Question 262

Which specially designed walking stick might provide comfort for permanent users or those with painful hands?

A. crook handle stick

B. Fischer stick

C. swan-necked shafted stick

D. T-shaped handle stick

E. wooden stick

Question 263

A late-middle-aged woman presents with chronic right hip and anterior thigh pain, with increased localised temperature. Lately she has needed a walking stick. During the past six months her relatives have noticed progressive hearing loss, as well as some facial changes, most notably enlargement of her mandible.

What would be a reasonable first-line investigation?

A. bone biopsy

B. bone-specific alkaline phosphatase

C. plain X-ray

D. serum procollagen 1 N-terminal peptide

E. serum 25-hydroxyvitamin D

Question 264

A 90-year-old man attends the emergency department following a fall. He complains of pain in his right hip area since the fall. He usually lives alone, mobilises with a stick indoors and three-wheeled walker outdoors. His past medical history includes hypertension, ischaemic heart disease and cardiac pacemaker insertion. On examination he complains of severe pain on internal and external rotation of the right hip. An X-ray of his hip does not demonstrate a fracture. Despite initial analgesia, he is unable to mobilise with the physiotherapy team due to pain in his right hip. What is the most appropriate next step?

A. CT scan of right hip

B. discharge to a temporary care home placement

C. MRI scan of right hip

D. repeat physiotherapy assessment after additional analgesia

E. repeat X-ray in two weeks

Question 265

An 84-year-old woman has broken her hip following a fall. The orthopaedic team have recommended she have surgical fixation as soon as possible. Her past medical history includes a non-ST elevation myocardial infarct nine months ago. Since then she has been taking aspirin and clopidogrel. What is the most appropriate advice to give to the surgical team?

A. a preoperative blood transfusion should be given

B. antiplatelets should be withheld and surgery should be delayed for at least five days

C. spinal or epidural anaesthesia techniques are preferable

D. surgery should occur as soon as possible

E. the risks of surgery outweigh the potential benefits at this time

Question 266

You have been invited to help write some local guidelines by the orthopaedic team to help improve the quality of care older people receive while having surgery for hip fractures. Which of the following is appropriate prior to surgery?

A. antibiotic prophylaxis

B. delay surgery until MRSA eradicated

C. do not operate at weekends

D. limb traction

E. routine echocardiography

Question 267

Regarding the use of low molecular weight heparin around the time of emergency hip surgery, which of the following statements about the commencement and duration is most accurate?

A. 6 hours after surgery and continued for 28 days

B. 6 hours after surgery and continued until independently mobile

C. 24 hours after surgery and continued for 14 days

D. 48 hours after surgery and continued for 28 days

E. just prior to surgery and continued until discharge

Question 268

You are asked to review an older person with a hip fracture who is due to go for surgical fixation. The anaesthetic team ask you what type of fracture has been sustained because they are curious as to what type of operation will be performed. Which of the following should be classified as an intracapsular fracture?

A. basal cervical

B. inter-trochanteric

C. per-trochanteric

D. subcapital

E. subtrochanteric

Question 269

When an 80-year-old woman was assessed in the community hospital, she was noted to have rheumatoid arthritis deformities involving her hands. She was very keen to return home as soon as feasible. She can weight bear through the length of their forearm rather than her hand or wrist. Which walking aid is most likely to be of benefit to her?

A. gutter frame

B. rollator frame

C. tripod walking stick

D. walking crutches

E. Zimmer frame

Stroke Care

LEARNING OBJECTIVE:

To assess patients presenting acutely with stroke and TIA, including suitability for cerebral reperfusion treatments and their subsequent ongoing medical management within an organised stroke service.

Areas to cover are:

- Epidemiology of stroke, particularly pertinent to older people, e.g. incidence, prevalence, disease burden.
- Definitions of stroke (including cerebral infarction and intracerebral haemorrhage), transient ischaemic attacks (TIAs) and transient focal neurological episodes (including relating to cerebral amyloid angiopathy [CAA]).

- Knowledge of neuroanatomy, physiology, blood supply and application of pathophysiology of these to common and rarer causes of TIA and stroke syndromes (e.g. thromboembolism, arterial dissection, cerebral venous sinus thrombosis, small vessel disease, CAA).
- An understanding of an accurate diagnosis of patients with suspected TIA or minor stroke including identification of relevant comorbidities,

vascular risk factors and lifestyle modification.

- Acute stroke and TIA management, e.g. risk stratification, knowledge of Oxford Community Stroke Project (OCSP or 'Bamford') classification, indicators for intravenous stroke thrombolysis, monitoring, management of physiological parameters in acute stroke, management of physiological parameters in acute stroke, initial monitoring to identify early complications such as dysphagia, indicators for specialist service (including neurosurgical) referral.

- Complications of stroke and their management: short term, e.g. DVT, pressure sores, respiratory and urinary infection, depression; long term, e.g. contractures, seizures, neuropathic pain.

- Physical, psychological and social impact of stroke on patients and carers.

- Primary and secondary prevention measures, particularly risk factor management appropriate to older people, e.g. when to consider treatment of hypertension, use of statins, use of anticoagulants and antiplatelet agents, appropriate use of brain imaging, vascular imaging and cardiac investigations.

- Recognition of conditions that 'mimic' TIA and stroke in the context of systemic disease (including focal seizure, migraine, functional neurological presentations) and how to effectively manage these or make an appropriate referral (including selection of appropriate investigations, treatments and advice relevant to the patient's age, comorbidities and clinical presentation).

- Assessment and management of common complications of stroke (including dysphagia, immobility, medical).

Questions

Question 270

A 78-year-old man presents to hospital following a right partial anterior circulation stroke. Despite appropriate thrombolysis intervention, he is left with a residual left-sided weakness of his arm and leg. At the time of discharge from hospital, he can mobilise independently with a four-wheeled walking frame but requires the assistance of a carer to help with washing and dressing. What is his current score on the modified Rankin scale?

A. 1
B. 2
C. 3
D. 4
E. 5

Question 271

An 83-year-old woman arrives in the emergency department three and a half hours after the sudden onset of right arm and face weakness and speech disturbance. A CT scan of her brain excludes intracerebral haemorrhage. Which of the following statements regarding thrombolysis for this woman's stroke is most likely to be correct?

A. an initial blood pressure reading above 185/110 mmHg excludes thrombolysis

B. antiplatelet drugs should not be given until at least 48 hours after thrombolysis

C. she should be assessed for suitability for intra-arterial clot extraction in preference to thrombolysis

D. thrombolysis is rarely indicated between three and four and a half hours after the onset of symptoms for people aged over 80

E. thrombolysis would not be indicated if she is currently taking apixaban

Question 272

A 71-year-old man has had a left total anterior circulation stroke and is currently receiving care on the stroke unit. He has dysphagia and cannot safely swallow enough to meet his nutritional needs. In which of the following situations would it be most appropriate to advocate percutaneous gastrostomy tube insertion?

A. clinical evidence of dehydration

B. high risk of sacral pressure ulceration

C. no improvement in swallow four weeks after stroke onset

D. palliative approach to care

E. requiring nasal bridle use to retain nasogastric tube

Question 273

You see a 77-year-old-woman in the neurovascular clinic and diagnose that she had a non-disabling stroke within the last 48 hours. Which of the following statements regarding future stroke prevention for her is correct?

A. atorvastatin should be offered if non-HDL cholesterol does not reduce following lifestyle advice

B. clopidogrel 300 mg should be given as soon as possible for people in sinus rhythm

C. do not change blood pressure medication until two weeks after symptom onset

D. target systolic blood pressure consistently below 140 mmHg

E. there is no need for brain imaging prior to starting anticoagulation for people in atrial fibrillation

Question 274

In the OCSP classification of subtypes of cerebral infarction, what is the definition of a 'lacunar infarct'?

A. a combination of new higher cerebral dysfunction (e.g. dysphasia), homonymous visual field defect and ipsilateral motor and/or sensory deficit of at least two areas (out of face, arm and leg)

B. a pure motor stroke, a pure sensory stroke, a sensori-motor stroke or an ataxic hemiparesis

C. any of ipsilateral cranial nerve palsy with contralateral motor and/or sensory deficit; bilateral motor and/or sensory deficit; disorder of conjugate eye movement; cerebellar dysfunction; isolated homonymous visual field defect

D. higher cerebral dysfunction alone or with a motor/sensory deficit confined to one limb

E. none of the above

Question 275

An 82-year-old man was admitted from his residential home with a history of sudden-onset of loss of consciousness. His medical history did not reveal any risk factors for intracerebral haemorrhage, such as systemic hypertension, recent trauma or use of medications, and there had been no history of any cognitive impairment. His blood pressure was 160/100 mmHg. He scored 8 (E2M4V2) on the Glasgow Coma Scale and had right-sided hemiplegia, bilateral extensor plantar responses and asymmetric pupillary reflexes. A cranial CT scan showed a 6 cm × 3 cm hematoma in the right occipital lobe causing midline shift, and a smaller cortical bleed in the left posterior frontal lobe. He subsequently died. A post mortem revealed a progressive accumulation of congophilic, immunoreactive, amyloid protein in the walls of small- to medium-sized arteries and arterioles predominantly located in the leptomeningeal space, cortex, and, to a lesser extent, in the capillaries and veins. What is the underlying diagnosis?

A. CADASIL

B. cerebral amyloid angiopathy

C. Fabry's disease

D. microbleeds

E. white matter hyperintensities

Question 276

An 82-year-old patient has no asymmetric facial, arm or leg weakness, no speech disturbance, no visual field deficit, but has experienced syncope. There has been no seizure activity. What would be his score on the ROSIER scale?

A. −2

B. −1

C. 0

D. 1

E. 2

Question 277

An 87-year-old woman develops pneumonia while recovering in hospital following a recent right partial anterior circulation stroke. Her swallow has been affected by the stroke, and she now receives a modified diet. Which of the following clinical features is associated with an increased risk of food aspiration while swallowing?

A. absence of cough during eating

B. chronic obstructive airway disease

C. current smoker

D. poor dental hygiene

E. requiring assistance with feeding

Question 278

A district hospital in a rural location is considering a business case for opening a specialist stroke unit. The number needed to treat on a specialist stroke unit to prevent one death, compared to non-specialist care, is likely to be closest to which figure?

A. 7

B. 15

C. 33

D. 75

E. 150

Question 279

A 77-year-old man on the stroke unit is six days into his recovery from a partial right anterior circulation infarct. He is currently mobile with the assistance of one person and still requires help with daily activities such as washing and dressing. The multidisciplinary team feel that he is a good candidate to be picked up by the local early supported discharge team. Which of the following is most likely to be correct regarding input from this type of team when compared to conventional inpatient rehabilitation?

A. greater financial costs

B. improved carer mood scores

C. improved patient subjective health status

D. lower patient dependency rates

E. reduced length of stay by an average of two days

Question 280

A 70-year-old right-handed retired academic is recovering from a left partial anterior circulation stroke, which has mainly affected her language ability. While talking she is able to form sentences quite well but struggles with certain words. This causes her to become very frustrated, and there are numerous phonemic paraphrasias contained within her speech. She is able to obey even complex verbal instructions and can read well but currently struggles with writing. It is notable that she is unable to accurately repeat even simple verbal phrases. Which is the best description of her pattern of aphasia?

A. anomic aphasia

B. Broca's (non-fluent) aphasia

C. conduction aphasia

D. global aphasia

E. Wernicke's (fluent) aphasia

Question 281

A 79-year-old man is receiving rehabilitation on the stroke unit following a left total anterior circulation stroke. Over the last few weeks he has developed increased tone in his right hand and arm. This has resulted in pain in his hand, and the ward staff report difficulty cleaning his palm on the affected side. Which of the following interventions would be most useful in this situation?

A. alcohol neurolysis

B. *Clostridium botulinum* toxin type A injections

C. functional electrical stimulation

D. oral tizanidine

E. wrist splinting

Question 282

A 76-year-old woman is admitted to the stroke unit following a left total anterior circulation infarct. This has caused a right hemiparesis, and she is currently only able to transfer with the assistance of two people. She is receiving a modified diet but is able to swallow tablets. She has no past medical history of note, but an admission ECG showed her to be in atrial fibrillation. Which of the following interventions is most appropriate to reduce the risk of developing venous thromboembolism in the first two weeks following the stroke for this woman?

A. a novel oral anticoagulant

B. above knee graduated pressure stockings

C. low molecular weight heparin injections

D. oral aspirin 300 mg daily

E. oral warfarin (INR target: 2.0 to 3.0)

Question 283

A 78-year-old man had a left carotid territory TIA the day before he is seen in the neurovascular clinic. His past medical history includes ischaemic heart disease, type 2 diabetes and COPD. He is mobile with a single walking stick and independent in daily activities. A carotid Doppler demonstrates a significant stenosis of his left carotid artery. Compared to carotid endarterectomy, which of the following factors is most beneficial for carotid artery stenting for symptomatic carotid artery stenosis?

A. does not require a general anaesthetic

B. greater reduction in risk of ipsilateral stroke between 30 days and five years post-procedure

C. lower risk of cranial nerve damage

D. lower risk of periprocedural death or stroke

E. peri-procedural risks are lower for people aged over 70 years

Question 284

A 70-year-old man has made a complete recovery from a left lacunar stroke and is being discharged home. He asks when he can safely return to having sexual intercourse. Which answer is correct?

A. as soon as he feels ready
B. his risk of stroke will be lowest if he permanently refrains
C. not until after his stroke clinic review appointment
D. once his systolic blood pressure is consistently below 130 mmHg
E. six weeks after his stroke

Question 285

A 90-year-old man is recovering following a left lacunar stroke. He has reduced movement of all muscle groups down his right-hand side. He complains of pain developing within his right shoulder. Which management strategy would be most useful for his shoulder pain?

A. electromyographic biofeedback
B. functional electrical stimulation
C. oral paracetamol
D. provision of an overhead pulley to his bed
E. strapping or a sling for his right arm

Question 286

A 77-year-old woman has been rehabilitating on the stroke unit for the last three weeks following a stroke. Recently her progress has been impaired by the development of uncontrollable tearful episodes. There is no clear trigger for these but they do seem more frequent when her friends and family visit the unit. She denies low mood but her oral intake has been noted to be quite low and she reports poor sleeping. She scored

22 out of 30 on the Montreal Cognitive Assessment test. Which of the following terms best describes her presentation?

A. anxiety
B. delirium
C. depression
D. emotionalism
E. vascular dementia

Question 287

A 63-year-old man presents with an acute onset of a right-sided weakness and aphasia within the last few hours. An initial CT scan excludes intracerebral haemorrhage, and a subsequent magnetic resonance angiogram shows a clot occluding a left-sided cerebral vessel. Which of the following is most likely to be correct regarding the use of mechanical clot retrieval devices for treating acute ischaemic stroke?

A. effective up to 12 hours after symptom onset
B. increased risk of haemorrhagic transformation
C. metallic objects, such as cardiac pacemakers, are contraindications
D. most effective for lacunar strokes
E. usually performed after intravenous thrombolysis

Question 288

You see a 91-year-old man in the neurovascular clinic. He describes having a right carotid artery territory TIA two days previously. His symptoms lasted around 30 minutes, and then he made a full recovery. He has not previously had any similar symptoms. Neurological examination does not reveal any residual deficit, and he scores well on a brief cognitive assessment. His ECG shows him to be in sinus rhythm. He is usually fully independent and asks when he can return to driving. Which answer is correct?

A. he can only return to driving if symptom-free for six months

B. he can return to driving immediately but needs to inform the DVLA

C. he needs to stop driving for one month and does not need to inform the DVLA

D. he should stop driving for three months and should inform the DVLA

E. he should stop driving permanently

Question 289

A 61-year-old right-handed smoker presents to the neurovascular clinic. He reports episodes of amnesia occurring around once a month over the last year. His partner says that during the episodes he continually asks questions, such as 'where am I?' or 'who are you?', but otherwise seems to function normally. After about 40 minutes he returns to his usual self. Sometimes the episodes are triggered by stressful events, but on other occasions have occurred when he first got up in the morning. He was made redundant two years ago and reports some financial pressure. He does not drink alcohol. No abnormalities are detected on physical and cognitive examinations. What is the most likely diagnosis for his recurrent symptoms?

A. functional amnesic state

B. transient amnesic epilepsy

C. transient global amnesia

D. transient ischaemic attack

E. urinary tract infection

Question 290

A 64-year-old woman is admitted to the hyperacute stroke unit with focal neurological symptoms. After initial evaluation, a functional disorder is suspected. Which of the following statements is most accurate regarding this diagnosis?

A. around 25% of people presenting to hyperacute stroke units have functional disorders

B. Hoover's sign has a high sensitivity but a low specificity

C. in around 90% of cases, the deficit resolves within a two-year follow-up period

D. normal MRI brain scanning, including DWI imaging, excludes acute stroke

E. suggested by isolated non-fluent aphasia

Question 291

A 72-year-old man reports some visual difficulties during your stroke round. On examination you note a left lower homonymous quadranopia. Where is his lesion?

A. left occipital lobe

B. left parietal lobe

C. pituitary gland

D. right occipital lobe

E. right parietal lobe

Tissue Viability

LEARNING OBJECTIVE:

To know how to assess, diagnose and monitor common types of leg and pressure ulceration and surgical and other wounds in older patients.

Areas to cover are:

- Basic biology and disease processes of ageing skin.
- Aetiology, risk factors and pathology of common causes of ulceration.
- Nutrition relating to tissue viability.
- Prevention of ulceration in particular pressure relief (e.g. knowledge of pressure-relieving and other specialist equipment and their uses).
- Assessment and diagnosis of common causes of skin ulceration (venous ulceration, pressure skin damage, diabetic foot, ulceration, lipodermatosclerosis, benign and malignant skin lesions, vasculitis).
- Risk scores (e.g. Waterlow, Norton, Braden) for prevention of pressure ulceration.
- Principles of wound and stump care.
- Management of ulceration and infection (including dressings, topical and systemic antibiotics, compression treatment, larval, vacuum therapy).
- Indications and techniques for non-surgical and surgical debridement.
- Diagnosis of benign or malignant lesions and reasons for non-healing.
- Indications for different dressings and other therapy.
- Unusual causes of non-healing, e.g. malignancy, vasculitis.

Questions

Question 292

A 73-year-old woman who has previously had a stroke is admitted to your ward. She is found to have a pressure ulcer on her sacrum at the time of admission. Which of the following treatment options is most likely to accelerate wound healing in the majority of older people with skin pressure ulceration?

A. a high specification foam mattress

B. negative pressure wound therapy

C. nutritional supplements

D. skin barrier creams

E. systemic antibiotics

Question 293

An 84-year-old man seen in your outpatient clinic has a long history of chronic bilateral venous leg ulceration. He also has severe arthritis of his left knee and has been told he could have joint replacement surgery once his ulceration has resolved. Which of the following pharmacological treatment options has the best evidence base for improving venous ulcer healing rates?

A. aspirin

B. mesoglycan

C. micronised purified flavonoid fraction

D. pentoxifylline

E. zinc

Question 294

In a residential home, an 83-year-old resident expresses concerns about a painful ulcer on the leg. A tissue viability nurse has been asked to help. The ulcer has a necrotic, devitalised, infected base. Which of the following intervention techniques would be most suitable?

A. autolytic debridement

B. mechanical debridement

C. scrubbing only

D. sharp debridement

E. topical antiseptics only

Question 295

A 70-year-old presents with two ulcers. One appears to be painful, especially when elevated, appearing as a punched out ulcer on the right little toe. It is covered with cold, white, shiny, hairless skin. A venous ulcer is also found on the left lower leg, above the medial malleolus. It is painless. Ankle-brachial pressure index <0.9, pulses reduced or absent. What is the appropriate management?

A. anti-microbial dressing

B. bacterial swabs

C. compression treatment

D. pentoxifylline

E. specialist vascular assessment

Question 296

An 84-year-old Caucasian female was transferred from an emergency department to a frailty assessment unit following a fall and fracturing her right distal femur. She had bilateral lower leg swelling, pain and erythema. In the emergency department she had been started on flucloxacillin for bilateral cellulitis. However, the blood results showed no evidence of active infection. Following the comprehensive geriatric assessment, the antibiotics were stopped, and the patient's condition was diagnosed as lipodermatosclerosis. What is the most appropriate management plan?

A. capsaicin

B. laser ablation

C. sclerotherapy

D. stanozolol

E. venous stasis using compression therapy and weight reduction

Question 297

The Waterlow score is a commonly used tool to estimate the risk of an adult developing pressure areas. Which of the following factors would score most highly?

A. aged 65 to 74 years old

B. breakdown on skin present

C. dual incontinence

D. paraplegic neurological deficit

E. restricted mobility

Question 298

An 89-year-old man is assessed for his risk of pressure ulceration at the time of hospital admission. He is judged to be at high risk due to a combination of cognitive impairment and reduced mobility to the extent that he cannot reposition himself. What would be a reasonable maximum time interval between ward staff changing his position?

A. one hour

B. two hours

C. four hours

D. six hours

E. eight hours

Question 299

An 85-year-old man is admitted onto a community rehabilitation ward following a prolonged stay with pneumonia. He had become immobile with hypoactive delirium, and subsequently physically deconditioned. During this period, he developed bilateral grade two pressure ulcers on his heels. Other pressure areas were intact. He is now able to transfer independently and mobilise a short distance with minimal assistance from one person. He was eating most of his small-sized meals, and his weight was stable.

TABLE 12.5

Investigations.

Ankle-brachial pressure indices (ABPI)	0.85 bilaterally

Which of the following is most important in managing his pressure ulcers overnight?

A. alternating pressure mattress

B. encourage him to sit out and practise mobilising

C. high protein diet

D. referral for arterial duplex ultrasound studies

E. referral to community tissue viability team

Question 300

A 90-year-old woman developed a mark on her sacrum while being treated for pneumonia. She had been using a continence pad. Examination showed a 3 cm by 2 cm area over the sacrum and loss of the dermis and blistering. It does not extend to the underlying fascia or bone. Which would be the appropriate classification?

A. grade one ulcer

B. grade two ulcer

C. grade three ulcer

D. grade four ulcer

E. moisture-associated skin damage

Answers for Chapter 12: Palliative care

229 Correct Answer: C

Explanation: The diagnosis is neutropenic sepsis. Early recognition and prompt treatment are paramount to avoid fatality. The patient should be managed as high-risk neutropenic sepsis. Specialist assessment and management in an acute hospital setting involves implementation of the UK Sepsis Trust 'Sepsis Six' bundle within the first hour following recognition of sepsis. Prompt administration of intravenous broad-spectrum antibiotics is mandatory. G-CSF (granulocyte colony-stimulating factor) should be considered in patients with a predicted prolonged neutropenia, after discussion with a haematologist or consultant oncologist. Passive immunisation with specific immunoglobulins may be useful in selected patients, e.g. varicella zoster immune globulin (VZIG) may be used for prophylaxis after contact with varicella zoster in the non-thrombocytopenic patient. In starting antibiotic therapy, according to current guidelines, beta lactam monotherapy with piperacillin with tazobactam as initial empiric antibiotic therapy should be offered to patients with suspected neutropenic sepsis who need intravenous treatment unless there are patient-specific or local microbiological contraindications. The guidelines specifically advise against offering an aminoglycoside, either as monotherapy or in dual therapy, for the initial empiric treatment of suspected neutropenic sepsis unless there are patient-specific or local microbiological indications.

Reading

Febrile Neutropenia in an Oncology Patient, 2014. www.pharmacytimes.com/publications/health-system-edition/2014/september2014/febrile-neutropenia-in-an-oncology-patient.

Neutropenic sepsis: Prevention and management in people with cancer. Clinical Guideline [CG151]. Published: 19 September 2012.

Walji N, Chan AK, Peake DR. Common acute oncological emergencies: Diagnosis, investigation and management. *Postgrad Med J* 2008; 84 (994): 418–427.

230 Correct Answer: E

Explanation: Patient-centred approaches to the deprescribing process have been proposed, but these can be difficult to implement due to fragmented care and the time-consuming process of documenting nuanced medication-related decisions—another reason cited as increasing inertia to deprescribing. Previous studies have identified that prescribing medicines with questionable benefits is common in nursing home residents. Deprescribing is not a new concept. Prescriber behaviours contribute to this (e.g. reluctance to stop medications started by other prescribers or specialists, devolved responsibility). Prescriptions for predominantly preventative drugs such as antihypertensives, anticoagulants, antiplatelets, statins and bisphosphonates all tend to increase in the years leading up to and following admission to the nursing home.

Reading

Welsh TJ, McGrogan A, Mitchell A. Deprescribing in the last years of life: it's hard to STOPP. *Age Ageing* 2020; afaa081.

231 Correct Answer: D

Explanation: Oramorph is effective in reducing symptoms of breathlessness, both against a background of end-stage COPD and end-stage cardiac failure. Breathlessness that persists at rest or on minimal exertion despite optimal treatment of the underlying disease(s) is termed 'refractory breathlessness'. Opioids have a growing evidence base for decreasing refractory breathlessness in advanced COPD. There is no evidence that benzodiazepines such as lorazepam relieve symptoms of breathlessness in COPD, and they carry significant risk of respiratory depression. As such, they should be avoided here. Glycopyrronium is an anticholinergic, which is an intervention of choice for excessive respiratory secretions in the end-of-life care setting, not indicated here. There is no indication that increasing inspired oxygen will relieve breathlessness here, and it may well drive carbon dioxide retention. Reassurance alone is inadequate, in this situation, for reducing the subjective experience of breathlessness.

232 Correct Answer: C

Explanation: As a general rule, one sixth of the total daily dose of regular opioid is prescribed to be taken when required for breakthrough pain. The opioid formulations most commonly used in the UK to treat breakthrough pain have a duration of action of approximately four hours. After administering a dose of breakthrough analgesic, the blood level of the opioid is, effectively, doubled for a short period, hopefully enabling pain control to be regained.

Reading

How to manage breakthrough pain. *Clinical Pharmacist*, 1 January 2009. Pharmaceutical journal. www.pharmaceutical-journal.com/careers-and-jobs/career-feature/how-to-manage-breakthrough-pain/10377845.article.

233 Correct Answer: A

Explanation: Metastatic spinal cord compression (MSCC) is defined as spinal cord or cauda equina compression by direct pressure and/or induction of vertebral collapse or instability by metastatic spread or direct extension of malignancy that threatens or causes neurological disability. MRI of the spine in patients with suspected MSCC should be supervised and reported by a radiologist and should include sagittal T1 and/or short T1 inversion recovery sequences of the whole spine, to prove or exclude the presence of spinal metastases. Sagittal T2 weighted sequences should also be performed to show the level and degree of compression of the cord or cauda equina by a soft tissue mass and to detect lesions within the cord itself. Consider myelography if other imaging modalities are contraindicated or inadequate. Myelography should only be undertaken at a neuroscience or spinal surgical centre because of the technical expertise required and because patients with MSCC may deteriorate following myelography and require urgent decompression. Plain radiographs of the spine are not performed, either to make or to exclude the diagnosis of spinal metastases or MSCC. In patients with a previous diagnosis of malignancy, routine MR imaging of the spine is not recommended if they are asymptomatic. Serial imaging of the spine in asymptomatic patients with cancer who are at high risk of developing spinal metastases should only be performed as part of a randomised controlled trial.

Reading

Metastatic spinal cord compression in adults: Risk assessment, diagnosis and management Clinical Guideline. Published: November 2008. www.nice. org.uk/guidance/cg75.

234 Correct Answer: C

Explanation: He is describing allodynia. Certain chemotherapy drugs are more likely to cause neuropathy. These include platinum drugs, such as oxaliplatin; taxanes, such as docetaxel; vinca alkaloids, such as vincristine; and myeloma treatments, such as bortezomib. According to current guidelines, patients should be offered a choice of amitriptyline, duloxetine, gabapentin or pregabalin as initial treatment for neuropathic pain (except trigeminal neuralgia). The guidelines also recommend that certain specific medications should not be used to treat neuropathic pain – apart from trigeminal neuralgia – in non-specialist settings, unless advised by a specialist to do so (see clause 1.1.12, pp. 11–12)

- Cannabis sativa extract
- Capsaicin patch

- Lacosamide
- Lamotrigine
- Levetiracetam
- Morphine
- Oxcarbazepine
- Topiramate

Reading

Brown TJ, Sedhom R, Gupta A. Chemotherapy-induced peripheral neuropathy. *JAMA Oncol* 2019; 5 (5): 750.
Neuropathic pain in adults: Pharmacological management in non-specialist settings. Clinical Guideline. Published: 20 November 2013. www.nice.org.uk/guidance/cg173.

235 Correct Answer: E

Explanation: Senna is an effective laxative. Evidence does not support docusate being a useful therapy. Patients are recommended to avoid:

- Phosphate enemas (if possible) as they can sometimes cause water and electrolyte disturbances, especially in people aged 65 years or older, and when comorbidities are present.
- Bulk-forming laxatives (e.g. bran, ispaghula), especially in opioid-induced constipation.
- Glycerol suppositories are unlikely to be effective.

Reading

Fakheri RJ, Volpicelli FM. Things we do for no reason: Prescribing docusate for constipation in hospitalized adults. *J Hosp Med* 2019; 14: 110–113.
NICE Constipation. Constipation, last revised in May 2020. https://cks.nice.org.uk/constipation#!scenario.

236 Correct Answer: D

Explanation: Dexamethasone oral 8 mg twice daily + omeprazole 20 mg daily is recommended.

Reading

Initial management of superior vena cava obstruction. https://handbook.ggcmedicines.org.uk/guidelines/respiratory-system/initial-management-of-superior-vena-cava-obstruction/.

237 Correct Answer: E

Explanation: Allopurinol is given as prophylaxis to prevent hyperuricaemia and associated renal failure. This is a xanthine oxidase inhibitor which prevents the production of uric acid. Patients with established tumour lysis syndrome and patients at very high risk of tumour lysis should be given rasburicase instead. This is a recombinant urate oxidase enzyme which catalyses the breakdown of uric acid. Rasburicase is derived from a cDNA code from a modified *Aspergillus flavus* strain and expressed in a modified yeast strain of *Saccharomyces cerevisiae*. A recombinant urate oxidase enzyme, rasburicase converts existing uric acid to allantoin, which is five to ten times more soluble in urine than uric acid. Rasburicase differs from allopurinol since it can affect existing plasma uric acid; allopurinol affects only the future production of uric acid by inhibiting xanthine oxidase.

Reading

Ueng S. Rasburicase (Elitek): A novel agent for tumor lysis syndrome. *Proc (Bayl Univ Med Cent)* 2005; 18 (3): 275–279.

238 Correct Answer E

Explanation: Technological development, for example of whole-body magnetic resonance imaging, made possible the adoption of new imaging modalities for a better approach for these patients. This imaging modality is helpful for staging, to gauge response assessment, and to the study of therapeutic changes in bone marrow. When metastatic spinal cord compression is suspected or confirmed, spinal stability must be assessed before any attempt is made to mobilise. Plain radiographs do not have a rôle in the investigation of suspected spinal cord compression. Requesting a lumbar spine MRI only is incorrect, as whole spine MRI is necessary as multi-level spinal metastases may occur. Further investigations are appropriate as she has metastatic cancer, even if she is receiving palliative care. Patients will not necessarily present with classic symptoms and signs; asymmetrical or unilateral signs are possible and only around 50% have a clinical sensory level.

Reading

Godinho MV, Lopes FPPL, Costa FM. Whole-body magnetic resonance imaging for the assessment of metastatic breast cancer. *Cancer Manag Res* 2018; 10: 6743–6756.

239 Correct Answer: E

Explanation: The patient has uncontrolled pain and yet is exhibiting symptoms suggestive of opioid side effects. These can occur due to non-opioid-responsive pain; for example, bone pain tends to be less responsive to opioids. Specialist advice regarding changing to an alternative opioid should be urgently sought. Complex pain and/or opioid-related side effects in patients with advanced disease are a clear indication for urgent advice and review by the specialist palliative care team. While amitriptyline is used for neuropathic pain, it is unlikely to be helpful for bone pain and would not be in the initial management. Although her pain is not controlled, increasing the morphine is likely to worsen her side effects, but stopping the morphine completely may well lead to escalating pain and withdrawal symptoms. Intravenous bisphosphonates are used for bone pain in metastatic cancer but should not be used acutely without assessing renal function, calcium and dental health.

240 Correct Answer: D

Explanation: The initial first-line treatment is rehydration. Monitor for fluid overload if there is renal impairment or in older people. Loop diuretics are rarely used and only if fluid overload develops; it is not effective for reducing serum calcium. After rehydration, consider intravenous bisphosphonates. May need to consider dialysis if severe renal failure.

SECOND LINE TREATMENTS:

- Glucocorticoids (inhibit 1,25OHD production).
- Calcimimetics.
- Calcitonin (can be considered if poor response to bisphosphonates; licensed for hypercalcaemia due to primary hyperparathyroidism, parathyroid carcinoma or renal failure).
- Parathyroidectomy (can be considered in acute presentation of primary hyperparathyroidism if severe hypercalcaemia and poor response to other measures).

Reading

Acute hypercalcaemia. www.rcem.ac.uk/docs/ External%20Guidance/10R.%20Acute%20 Hypercalcaemia%20-%20Emergency%20Guidance %20(Society%20for%20Endocrinology,%20 Jan%202014).pdf.

241 Correct Answer: C

Explanation: General indicators of decline include:

- General physical decline, increasing dependence and need for support.
- Repeated unplanned hospital admissions.
- Advanced disease—unstable, deteriorating, complex symptom burden.
- Presence of significant multi-morbidities.
- Decreasing activity—functional performance status declining (e.g. Barthel score) limited self-care, in bed or chair 50% of day and increasing dependence in most activities of daily living.
- Decreasing response to treatments, decreasing reversibility.
- Patient choice for no further active treatment and to focus on quality of life.
- Progressive weight loss (>10%) in past six months.
- A sentinel event, e.g. serious fall, bereavement, transfer to nursing home.
- Serum albumin <25 g/L.
- Considered eligible for DS1500 payment.

Reading

The Gold Standards Framework Proactive Identification Guidance (PIG), Gold Standards Framework/RCGP. www.goldstandardsframework.org.uk/cd-content/ uploads/files/PIG/NEW%20PIG%20-%20%20 %2020.1.17%20KT%20vs17.pdf.

242 Correct Answer: B

Explanation: The ReSPECT process recommendations are created through conversations between a person, their family and their healthcare professionals to understand what matters to them and what is realistic in terms of their care and treatment. Patient preferences and clinical recommendations are recorded on a non-legally-binding form which can be reviewed and adapted if circumstances change. The ReSPECT process can be for anyone but will have increasing relevance for people who have complex health needs, people who are likely to be nearing the end of their lives, and people who are at risk of sudden deterioration or cardiac arrest. Some people will want to record their care and treatment preferences for other reasons.

Reading

www.resus.org.uk/respect.

243 Correct Answer: C

Explanation: If a patient with capacity refuses CPR, or a patient lacking capacity has a valid and applicable advance decision to refuse treatment, specifically refusing CPR, this must be respected. If the healthcare team is as certain as it can be that a person is dying as an inevitable result of underlying disease or a catastrophic health event, and CPR would not restart the heart and breathing for a sustained period, CPR should not be attempted. Where a patient or those close to a patient disagree with a DNACPR decision, a second opinion should be offered. Even when CPR has no realistic prospect of success, there must be a presumption in favour of explaining the need and basis for a DNACPR decision to a patient, or to those close to a patient who lacks capacity. A DNACPR decision does not override clinical judgement in the unlikely event of a reversible cause of the person's respiratory or cardiac arrest that does not match the circumstances envisaged when that decision was made and recorded.

Reading

Decisions relating to cardiopulmonary resuscitation: Guidance from the British Medical Association, the Resuscitation Council (UK) and the Royal College of Nursing (previously known as the 'Joint Statement') (Third edition) (1st revision), 2016. www.resus. org.uk/sites/default/files/2020-05/20160123%20 Decisions%20Relating%20to%20CPR%20-%20 2016.pdf.

Answers for Chapter 12: Psychiatry of old age

244 Correct Answer: C

Explanation: The best scientific evidence currently exists for the use of home-based non-pharmacological behavioural management techniques, carer-based interventions, including psychoeducation for patients and carers. It is worth noting that certain pharmacological interventions are not recommended. Tricyclic antidepressants are not recommended because of their anticholinergic adverse events. Haloperidol may be considered in the treatment of psychosis related to delirium superimposed on dementia, but it is not recommended for a different use in dementia. Although carbamazepine shows some benefit for agitation in dementia, mood stabilisers are often associated with severe side effects. Repeated transcranial magnetic stimulation may become a useful method, but the study of this method to treat behavioural and psychological symptoms of dementia (BPSD) is still in its infancy.

Reading

Cohen-Mansfield J, Jensen B. Assessment and treatment approaches for behavioral disturbances associated with dementia in the nursing home: Self-reports of physicians' practices. *J Am Med Dir Assoc* 2008; 9 (6): 406–413.
Tible OP, Riese F, Savaskan E, et al. Best practice in the management of behavioural and psychological symptoms of dementia. *Ther Adv Neurol Disord* 2017; 10 (8): 297–309.

245 Correct Answer: B

Explanation: Charles Bonnet syndrome (CBS) occurs predominantly in older, visually impaired people. Some experience complex visual hallucinations, but most experience elementary visual phenomena. CBS is associated with diseases affecting the retina, light transmission within the eye (e.g. cataract, corneal opacity) or visual pathways and visual cortex. Typical symptoms include simple hallucinations (colours and elementary shapes) geometrical patterns, disembodied faces and costumed figures. CBS is considered to be underreported due to patients' fears of being categorised as mentally ill. An important part of the management of CBS is an explanation and reassurance that the hallucinations are benign and harmless and do not signify mental illness. There is some case-report evidence for treatment with certain pharmacological agents, but currently none can be recommended for routine clinical use without further evidence for their efficacy.

Reading

Best J, Liu PY, Ffytche D, et al. Think sight loss, think Charles Bonnet syndrome. *Ther Adv Ophthalmol* 2019; 11: 2515841419895909.

Jacob A, Prasad S, Boggild M, et al. Charles Bonnet syndrome: elderly people and visual hallucinations. *BMJ* 2004; 328 (7455): 1552–1554.

Kennard C. Charles Bonnet syndrome—disturbing 'playthings of the brain'. *Pract Neurol* 2018; 18 (6): 434–435.

O'Brien J, Taylor JP, Ballard C, et al. Visual hallucinations in neurological and ophthalmological disease: Pathophysiology and management. *J Neurol Neurosurg Psychiatry* 2020; 91 (5): 512–519.

246 Correct Answer: D

Explanation: The history is too long for delirium. There is no longstanding cognitive impairment, so dementia is unlikely. There is no history of squalor, making Diogenes syndrome unlikely.

The likely diagnosis is dissociative fugue. Dissociative fugue is characterised by the sudden, unexpected travel away from home or one's customary place of daily activities, with inability to recall some or all of one's past. There can be confusion about personal identity. On occasion, patients assume a new identity. People suffering from fugue states appear normal to the lay observer. Patients usually exhibit no signs of psychopathology or cognitive deficit. Fugue patients differ from those with dissociative amnesia in that the former are usually unaware of their amnesia. Only upon resumption of their former identities do they recall past memories, at which time they usually become amnestic for experiences during the fugue episode. Often, patients suffering from fugue states take on an entirely new (and often unrelated) identity and occupation. Not much is known regarding the aetiology of this disorder. Clinical data suggest that predisposing factors include extreme psychosocial stress such as war or natural and human-made disasters, personal and/or financial pressures or losses, heavy alcohol use, and intense and overwhelming stress such as assault or rape. Personal identity is usually retained in transient global amnesia.

Reading

Maldonado, JR; Spiegel D (2008). "Dissociative disorders—Dissociative identity disorder (Multiple personality disorder)". In Hales RE; Yudofsky SC; Gabbard GO (eds.). *The American Psychiatric Publishing textbook of psychiatry* (5th ed.). Washington, DC: American Psychiatric Pub. pp. 681–710. ISBN 978-1-58562-257-3.

247 Correct Answer: A

Explanation: 'Anton's syndrome' describes the condition in which patients deny their blindness despite objective evidence of visual loss and moreover confabulate to support their stance. It is a rare extension of cortical blindness in which, in addition to the injury to the occipital cortex, other cortical centres are also affected, with patients typically behaving as if they were sighted. A suspicion of cortical blindness and Anton's syndrome should be considered in patients with atypical visual loss and evidence of occipital lobe injury. Cerebrovascular disease is the most common cause of Anton's syndrome, but any condition that may result in cortical blindness can potentially lead to Anton's syndrome. Management in these circumstances should accordingly focus on secondary prevention and rehabilitation. Cortically blind patients can potentially maintain perception to hand movements. This is described as the Riddoch phenomenon, when moving objects are visible but static objects are not.

Reading

Anton syndrome. https://eyewiki.aao.org/Anton_Syndrome.
Maddula M, Lutton S, Keegan B. Anton's syndrome due to cerebrovascular disease: A case report. *J Med Case Rep* 2009; 3: 9028. Published: 9 September 2009.

248 Correct Answer: C

Explanation: The symptoms started with personality change, making Alzheimer's disease unlikely. The history is too long for delirium. The nature of the history make dissociative fugue and transient global amnesia unlikely. Diogenes syndrome is a behavioural disorder described in the clinical literature in older individuals: the classical constellation of symptoms of this condition include extreme neglected physical state, social isolation, domestic squalor and tendency to hoard excessively (*syllogomania*). The spectrum of Diogenes syndrome in patients

with the behavioural variant of frontotemporal dementia includes a decline in self-awareness and self-care and collecting behaviour leading to a tendency for clutter in the living environment. Common to these patients tends to be a lack of insight. Also observed in these patients were prominent compulsive behaviours. Distinct from hoarding syndrome, most patients displayed little interest in the accumulated items once collected and were able to allow others to discard them without distress.

Reading

Cipriani G, Lucetti C, Vedovello M, Nuti A. Diogenes syndrome in patients suffering from dementia. *Dialogues Clin Neurosci* 2012; 14 (4): 455–460.
Finney CM, Mendez MF. Diogenes syndrome in frontotemporal dementia. *Am J Alzheimer's Dis Other Dementias* 2017; 438–443.

249 Correct Answer: D

Explanation: The description given is of the Montgomery and Åsberg depression rating scale (MADRS). The HADS is a self-rating scale. PHQ-9 is a self-reported depression assessment tool scoring each of the nine DSM-IV criteria as zero (not at all) to three (nearly every day). The Cornell scale is suitable for patients with cognitive deficit, not diagnostic for depression, but higher scores indicate greater need for further evaluation. The GDS has been specifically developed for use in geriatric patients; contains fewer somatic items; is suitable only for patients with no, mild, or moderate cognitive impairment (i.e. >15/30 on mini-mental state examination). It is well validated in older people, with a cut-off score in population over 60 of ≥5 suggesting depression.

Reading

Rodda J, Walker Z, Carter J. Depression in older adults. *BMJ* 2011; 343: d5219.

250 Correct Answer: D

Explanation: The presentation of older people with alcohol use disorders may be atypical (such as falls, confusion, depression) or masked by comorbid physical or psychiatric illness, which makes detection more difficult. Diagnostic criteria and screening instruments tend to focus on current levels of alcohol intake. The prevalence of alcohol misuse disorders in older people is generally accepted to be lower than in younger people. The ageing of populations worldwide means that the absolute number of older people with alcohol use disorders is on the increase. Finally, older people may be less likely than younger people to encounter the social, legal and occupational complications associated with alcohol use disorders.

Reading

O'Connell H, Chin AV, Cunningham C, Lawlor B. Alcohol use disorders in elderly people: Redefining an age old problem in old age. *BMJ* 2003; 327 (7416): 664–667.

251 Correct Answer: C

Explanation: Elder abuse can be categorised into being physical, psychological, sexual or financial exploitation and abuse secondary to neglect, with overlap existing between these categories. Physical elder abuse is associated with significant morbidity and mortality, as well as having a significant economic impact. The other options do not fit the description.

Reading

Pereira C, Fertleman M. Elder abuse: A common problem, commonly missed in trauma and orthopaedics. *Eur Geriatr Med* 2019; 10: 839–841.

252 Correct Answer: A

Explanation: The diagnosis is Charles Bonnet syndrome. Cataract surgery can improve symptoms in such patients.

Reading

Jefferis JM, Clarke MP, Taylor JP. Effect of cataract surgery on cognition, mood, and visual hallucinations in older adults. *J Cataract Refract Surg* 2015; 41 (6): 1241–1247.

253 Correct Answer: E

Explanation: There are ethical issues and issues of compliance. Notwithstanding, mobile phone/GPS technology has been seriously considered as assistive technology devices in this context.

Reading

Miskelly F. Electronic tracking of patients with dementia and wandering using mobile phone technology. *Age Ageing* 2005; 34 (5): 497–499.

254 Correct Answer: B

Explanation: The Protection of Vulnerable Adults (POVA) process should aim to establish all the facts, including that his daughter does indeed hold a lasting power of attorney. All POVA teams work to ensure that vulnerable adults are protected from abuse and neglect, and when a referral is received it may be necessary to act to keep individuals safe from further actual harm or risk of harm. When an allegation of abuse or neglect is received, a designated senior officer will coordinate the investigation. The investigation should also prompt subsequent safeguarding measures for the patient whilst she is on the ward, including managing subsequent meals and visits. It may also lead to a separate assessment of her husband and establish his diagnoses/needs. Some/all of the other options might subsequently be relevant but under the umbrella of the POVA process.

Answers for Chapter 12: Osteoporosis and Orthogeriatrics

255 Correct Answer: D

Explanation: The presence of a low-trauma vertebral fracture in a patient on long-term corticosteroids is an indication to start a bisphosphonate. Calcium and vitamin D alone are unlikely to be effective. Kyphoplasty is sometimes considered in people with symptoms beyond six weeks of the fracture but supportive evidence of efficacy is weak. It may be helpful to obtain a bone density scan in order to monitor the effect of treatment, but that can be arranged after starting treatment.

256 Correct Answer: D

Explanation: The fracture is associated with minimal or no trauma, as in a fall from standing height or less.

This is major criterion, along with others:

- The fracture line originates at the lateral cortex and is substantially transverse in its orientation, although it may become oblique as it progresses medially across the femur.
- Complete fractures extend through both cortices and may be associated with a medial spike; incomplete fractures involve only the lateral cortex.
- The fracture is non-comminuted or minimally comminuted.
- Localised periosteal or endosteal thickening of the lateral cortex is present at the fracture site ('beaking' or 'flaring').

Reading

Saita Y, Ishijima M, Kaneko K. Atypical femoral fractures and bisphosphonate use: Current evidence and clinical implications. *Ther Adv Chronic Dis* 2015; 6 (4): 185–193.

257 Correct Answer: D

Explanation: NICE guidelines recommend a bisphosphonate as initial therapy for osteoporosis. Risedronate is given weekly. If it is not tolerated because of the history of reflux disease, then monthly bisphosphonates, injectable bisphosphonates or denosumab are potential alternatives. Denosumab is recommended by NICE where bisphosphonates are not tolerated and there is an indication of more severe osteoporosis (T score < −3.5). Given this patient has already had a fracture and proven osteoporosis, it is not appropriate to continue calcium and vitamin D only because she has significant ongoing fracture risk. Raloxifene is a selective oestrogen receptor modulator. It is less effective as a treatment for osteoporosis compared to a bisphosphonate and is associated with an increased risk of venous thromboembolism. Teriparatide is an injectable parathyroid hormone analogue, and its main use is as a bone-building agent for patients with severe osteoporosis. Its administration as a daily injectable means that it is unsuitable for most patients.

258 Correct Answer: A

Explanation: Risk factors for osteoporosis

Independent of bone mineral density
   Age
   Previous fragility fracture
   Parental history of hip fracture
   Oral corticosteroid therapy (dependent on the dose and duration of treatment)
      Current smoking
   Alcohol intake ≥ three units/day
   Rheumatoid arthritis and other inflammatory arthropathies
   Body mass index ≤ 19
   History of falls
   Smoking

(Continued)

Explanation: Risk factors for osteoporosis
(Continued)

Depending on bone mineral density
  Untreated hypogonadism
  Malabsorption (e.g. Crohn's disease,
  ulcerative colitis, pancreatisis, coeliac disease)
  Endocrine disease (e.g. diabetes mellitus,
  hyperthyroidism, hyperparathyroidism)
  Chronic renal disease
  Chronic liver disease
  Chronic obstructive pulmonary disease
  Immobility
  Drugs (aromatase inhibitors, androgen
  deprivation therapy)

Reading

Poole KE, Compston JE. Osteoporosis and its management. *BMJ* 2006; 333 (7581): 1251–1256.

NICE, CKS. Osteoporosis – prevention of fragility fractures: What are the risk factors? https://cks.nice.org.uk/topics/osteoporosis-prevention-of-fragility-fractures/background-information/risk-factors/.

259 Correct Answer: A

Explanation: Denosumab is a fully human IgG2 monoclonal antibody that binds with high affinity to human RANKL and blocks binding of RANKL to RANK. Osteoprotegerin (OPG) is the natural inhibitor of RANKL. RANK and RANKL are expressed by endothelial cells and lymphocytes. ONJ is associated with oncology-dose parenteral antiresorptive therapy of bisphosphonates and denosumab.

Reading

Khan AA, Morrison A, Hanley DA, et al. Diagnosis and management of osteonecrosis of the jaw: A systematic review and international consensus. *J Bone Miner Res* 2015; 30 (1): 3–23.

McClung M. Rôle of RANKL inhibition in osteoporosis. *Arthritis Res Ther* 2007; 9 (Suppl 1): S3.

260 Correct Answer: B

Explanation: This patient's decreased vitamin D levels are secondary to a combination of poor dietary intake, decreased sunlight exposure and long-term anticonvulsant use. This led to hypocalcaemia precipitating a seizure and resultant bilateral femoral neck fractures secondary to decreased bone mineral density. Renal dysfunction may have potentiated these findings; however, it is unlikely to have been a major contributor to the acute presentation of seizure and hypocalcaemia. Bilateral neck of femur fractures can occur as a result of high impact trauma. Occurrence has been reported previously, secondary to electroconvulsive and pharmaco-convulsive therapy; however, it has become less prevalent since the initiation of the use of muscle relaxants during these procedures.

Reading

Rokan Z, Kealey WD. Osteomalacia: A forgotten cause of fractures in the elderly. *BMJ Case Rep* 2015; 2015: bcr2014207184.

261 Correct Answer: D

Approximate proportions:

- Upper GI symptoms (7%–47%)
- Acute phase response with first infusion (12%–42%)
- Hypocalcaemia (<1%)
- Nephrotoxicity (0%–0.6%)
- Osteonecrosis of the jaw (0.001%–0.067%)

Reading

Maraka S, Kennel KA. Bisphosphonates for the prevention and treatment of osteoporosis. *BMJ* 2015; 351: h3783.

262 Correct Answer: B

Explanation: Contoured handles, sometimes called Fischer sticks, are anatomically shaped handles which spread the pressure over a wider area of the palm to improve comfort for permanent users or those with painful hands, perhaps due to arthritis.

Reading

Disability Living Foundation. Choosing walking equipment. www.dlf.org.uk/factsheets/walking.

263 Correct Answer: C

Explanation: Plain X-ray is central to the evaluation of Paget's disease. X-rays are performed in all patients at the initial stage of evaluation. The radiographs of pagetoid bone have a classical appearance. Bone-specific alkaline phosphatase is a more sensitive blood test for diagnosis and can also be used as an index for treatment response, but availability may be limited. Serum 25-hydroxyvitamin D is measured to exclude osteomalacia as an alternative cause of an elevated alkaline phosphatase. Serum 25-hydroxyvitamin D is normal in Paget's disease. Serum procollagen 1 N-terminal peptide (P1NP, the amino-terminal propeptide of type 1 collagen) is a specific measure of bone formation that correlates well with activity on bone scintigraphy, but availability may be limited and/or cost prohibitive. The most sensitive and specific test for diagnosis is bone biopsy, but this is rarely needed. In weightbearing long bones such as the femur, diagnostic biopsy should be avoided because of the risk of fracture in an already compromised bone.

264 Correct Answer: A

Explanation: When there is a high suspicion of hip fracture, despite initial X-ray not showing a break, then an MRI scan is the recommended next test. However, this scan technique is not always rapidly available and can be contraindicated (e.g. cardiac pacemaker). NICE recommend the next best test is a CT scan. Repeat X-ray imaging at 24 to 48 hours is an option, but such a strategy would delay access to surgery, with resultant risks, in such a situation of high clinical suspicion of fracture.

Reading

National Institute for Health and Care Excellence. Hip fracture: Management. 2011. www.nice.org.uk/guidance/cgl24.
Scottish Intercollegiate Guidelines Network. Management of hip fracture in older people: A national clinical guideline, 2009. www.sign.ac.uk/sign-111-management-of-hip-fracture-in-older-people.

265 Correct Answer: D

Explanation: Elective surgery should be delayed for at least five days following withholding antiplatelets, but these drugs should not delay emergency surgery. Spinal or epidural anaesthesia is not recommended while on dual anti-platelet therapy. General anaesthesia is recommended.

Reading

Scottish Intercollegiate Guidelines Network. Management of hip fracture in older people: A national clinical guideline, 2009. www.sign.ac.uk/sign-111-management-of-hip-fracture-in-older-people.

266 Correct Answer: A

Explanation: Antibiotic prophylaxis is recommended prior to emergency hip surgery. Surgery should not be delayed by weekends or MRSA status. Limb traction is not helpful. Echocardiography would only be performed when there is a clinical indication.

Reading

Scottish Intercollegiate Guidelines Network. Management of hip fracture in older people: A national clinical guideline, 2009. www.sign.ac.uk/sign-111-management-of-hip-fracture-in-older-people.

267 Correct Answer: A

Explanation: Low molecular weight heparin (LMWH) is usually given six hours after surgery and continued for 28 days. LMWH can increase the risk of vertebral canal haematoma following spinal or epidural anaesthesia and such techniques are usually delayed until 10–12 hours after LMWH administration.

Reading

Scottish Intercollegiate Guidelines Network. Management of hip fracture in older people: A national clinical guideline, 2009. www.sign.ac.uk/sign-111-management-of-hip-fracture-in-older-people.

268 Correct Answer: D

Explanation: Subcapital and transcervical fractures are classified as intracapsular, and subdivided into undisplaced or displaced. Extracapsular fractures include per-, inter- and subtrochanteric locations. Basal cervical fractures lie on the intra- and extracapsular divide. They are usually considered as extracapsular in terms of prognosis and management.

For undisplaced intracapsular fractures, surgery allows early mobilisation and prevents delayed displacement. Internal fixation is recommended for most people. For displaced intracapsular fractures, hemiarthoplasty gives good results up to three years (typically preferred when shorter life expectancy). Total hip replacement may have benefits beyond three years but at an increased risk of early dislocation. The majority of extracapsular fractures are treated surgically with sliding hip screws.

Reading

Scottish Intercollegiate Guidelines Network. Management of hip fracture in older people: A national clinical guideline, 2009. www.sign. ac.uk/sign-111-management-of-hip-fracture-in-older-people.

269 Correct Answer: A

Explanation: Gutter frames have forearm troughs or 'gutters' that allow weight bearing through the forearm in patients who are unable to use the wrist or hand.

Reading

Disability Living Foundation. Choosing walking equipment. www.dlf.org.uk/factsheets/walking.

Answers for Chapter 12: Stroke

270 Correct Answer: C

Explanation: modified Rankin scale:

- Asymptomatic.
- Mild symptoms, no disability.
- Mild disability but independent with personal care.
- Moderate disability, independent mobility but requires help with personal care.
- Moderate disability, some assistance needed for mobility and personal care.
- Severe disability, immobile and requiring help with all care.
- Dead.

Reading

Modified Rankin Scale, https://www.mdcalc.com/modified-rankin-scale-neurologic-disability.

271 Correct Answer: E

Explanation: The balance of risks and benefits for thrombolysis is less clear for people aged over 80 when given between three and four and a half hours after symptom onset. It is recommended that an individual decision be made but thrombolysis would often still be appropriate. An initial blood pressure above 185/110 mmHg should have an attempt made to lower it to reduce the risk of haemorrhagic complications with thrombolysis. The current use of a novel oral anticoagulant or NOAC (e.g. apixaban) would usually exclude giving thrombolysis (dabigatran may be the exception as its effects can be rapidly reversed). Antiplatelet agents, unless haemorrhage is detected on repeat brain imaging or contraindicated for other reasons, are started 24 hours after thrombolysis. A combination of intravenous thrombolysis and intra-arterial clot extraction may be suitable for people with a proximal intracranial large vessel occlusion causing a disabling neurological deficit (National Institutes of Health Stroke Scale score of 6 or more) if the intra-arterial procedure can begin within five hours of symptom onset (the time window may extend to 24 hours in some circumstances). Thrombectomy would only be used alone in patients meeting the above criteria but with a contraindication to receiving thrombolysis.

Reading

Intercollegiate Stroke Working Party. *National clinical guideline for stroke* (Fifth edition), 2016.

272 Correct Answer: C

Explanation: Nasogastric tube insertion should be considered within 24 hours of presentation for acute stroke when oral intake is unsafe or inadequate. A switch to gastrostomy feeding should be considered when a nasogastric tune cannot be retained or tolerated despite trying a nasal bridle, or if swallowing has not improved by four weeks after stroke onset.

Reading

Intercollegiate Stroke Working Party. *National clinical guideline for stroke* (Fifth edition), 2016. London: Royal College of Physicians. https://www.rcplondon.ac.uk/guidelines-policy/stroke-guidelines. Also available at https://www.strokeaudit.org/SupportFiles/Documents/Guidelines/2016-National-Clinical-Guideline-for-Stroke-5t-(1).aspx

273 Correct Answer: B

Explanation: Atorvastatin (20–80 mg) is recommended for all people having had an ischaemic stroke or TIA. Clopidogrel 300 mg initially followed by 75 mg daily is recommended for people in sinus rhythm. Systolic blood pressure target should be consistently better than 130 mmHg for most people. Blood pressure lowering medication can be started immediately, when required, for people who have had a non-disabling stroke (recommendation to start after two weeks or at the point of hospital discharge, whichever comes sooner, for people who have had a disabling stroke). Brain imaging is recommended to exclude haemorrhage prior to starting anticoagulation for atrial fibrillation in all people who had had a cerebrovascular event.

Reading

Intercollegiate Stroke Working Party. *National clinical guideline for stroke* (Fifth edition), 2016. London: Royal College of Physicians. https://www.rcplondon.ac.uk/guidelines-policy/stroke-guidelines. Also available at https://www.strokeaudit.org/SupportFiles/Documents/Guidelines/2016-National-Clinical-Guideline-for-Stroke-5t-(1).aspx

274 Correct Answer: B

Explanation: A, C and D are definitions of total anterior circulation infarcts (TACI), partial anterior circulation infarcts (PACI) and posterior circulation infarcts (POCI), respectively.

Reading

Bamford J, Sandercock P, Dennis M, Burn J, Warlow C. Classification and natural history of clinically identifiable subtypes of cerebral infarction. *Lancet* 1991; 337: 1521–1526.

275 Correct Answer: B

Explanation: Cerebral amyloid angiopathy (CAA) is the dominant cause of lobar intracerebral haemorrhage in older people. Not only does it result in stroke and cognitive impairment in a significant proportion, but it is also an important component of the senile plaques found in people with Alzheimer's disease.

Reading

Banerjee G, Carare R, Cordonnier C, et al. The increasing impact of cerebral amyloid angiopathy: Essential new insights for clinical practice. *J Neurol Neurosurg Psychiatr* 2017; 88: 982–994.

Li Q, Yang Y, Reis C, et al. Cerebral small vessel disease. *Cell Transplant* 2018; 27 (12): 1711–1722.

Panicker JN, Nagaraja D, Chickabasaviah YT. Cerebral amyloid angiopathy: A clinicopathological study of three cases. *Ann Indian Acad Neurol* 2010; 13 (3): 216–220.

276 Correct Answer: B

Explanation: The ROSIER scale has been found to be effective in the initial differentiation of acute stroke from stroke mimics in the emergency department.

TABLE 12.6

'ROSIER' scale.

Has there been loss of consciousness or syncope?	−1
Has there been seizure activity?	−1
Is there a NEW ACUTE onset (or an awakening from sleep)	
1. Asymmetric facial weakness	1
2. Asymmetric arm weakness	1
3. Asymmetric leg weakness	1
4. Speech disturbance	1
5. Visual field defect	1

Reading

Nor AM, Davis J, Sen B, et al. The Recognition of Stroke in the Emergency Room (ROSIER) scale: Development and validation of a stroke recognition instrument. *Lancet Neurol* 2005; 4 (11): 727–734.

277 Correct Answer: E

Explanation: The absence of a cough while eating is normal; however, a lack of cough can occur in people who aspirate (e.g. seen during video fluoroscopic assessments). People requiring assistance with feeding are at a higher risk of aspirating. Aspiration increases the risk of developing pneumonia. Pneumonia is also more likely to develop when poor dental hygiene, current smoking and a history of COPD are present, but these factors probably do not increase the risk of aspiration per se. Aspiration risk is also elevated with reduced conscious level, wet/hoarse voice, weak cough mechanism, prolonged pharyngeal transit time and some medications (e.g. antipsychotics).

Reading

Scottish Intercollegiate Guidelines Network. Management of patients with stroke: Identification and management of dysphagia. National Clinical Guideline 119, 2010. www.sign.ac.uk/assets/sign119.pdf.

278 Correct Answer: C

Explanation: Studies suggest the number needed to treat (NNT) to prevent one death is 33; the NNT for one extra person returning to their own home is 20, but the confidence intervals are wide on these estimates. The benefit is most likely on units that provide several weeks of rehabilitation with specialist multidisciplinary teams rather than short stay units. This is probably true for people of all ages.

Reading

Scottish Intercollegiate Guidelines Network. Management of patients with stroke: Rehabilitation, prevention and management of complications, and discharge planning. National Clinical Guideline 118, 2010. www.sign.ac.uk/assets/sign118.pdf.

279 Correct Answer: D

Explanation: Early supported discharge teams benefit selected patients recovering from mild to moderate stroke. Evidence suggests improved independent survival rates and reduced length of stay by an average of eight days. They have not been shown to have an effect on patient mood or subjective health status, or carer mood or satisfaction. Financial costs are probably lower than those of conventional care. They are best if delivered by a dedicated multidisciplinary team. It is unclear if this model is applicable to very remote and rural locations.

Reading

Langhorne P, Holmqvist LW, Early supported discharge trialists. Early supported discharge after stroke. *J Rehabil Med* 2007; 39: 103–108.

280 Correct Answer: C

Explanation: Broca's (non-fluent) aphasia is caused by a lesion affecting the inferior frontal gyrus of the dominant hemisphere. There is reduced speech output typically in a stop-start/telegraphic pattern, difficulty articulating and an omission of verbs and prepositions from sentences. Those affected are able to understand speech and usually can read but not write. Speech repetition is impaired.

Transcortical motor aphasia is similar to Broca's aphasia, but those affected are still able to repeat phrases.

Wernicke's (fluent) aphasia is caused by lesions affecting the posterior superior lobe of the temporal lobe on the dominant side. This mainly limits comprehension of speech but production will also be abnormal in terms of sentence structure and word use. Repetition, reading and writing abilities are also affected.

Transcortical sensory aphasia is similar to Wernicke's aphasia, but those affected are still able to repeat phrases.

Anomic aphasia is a milder form of aphasia affecting Wernicke's area, resulting in difficulty finding some words, causing circumlocution and evident frustration. There is good understanding of speech, and those affected can usually read well but have the same word-finding problems when writing. Repetition is unaffected.

Conduction aphasia is similar to anomic aphasia, but those affected cannot repeat phrases. It is thought to be caused by damage to the arcuate fasciculus that connects Broca's and Wernicke's areas.

Global aphasia is the most severe form of speech disturbance due to a combination of lesions affecting Broca's and Wernicke's areas. Those affected express few words, have little comprehension and can't read or write.

Mixed non-fluent aphasia is a term for a less severe form of a combined Broca's and Wernicke's deficit, where expression and comprehension are both partially impaired. Paraphrasias are word errors, which can be semantic (e.g. 'apple' instead of 'orange') or phonemic.

281 Correct Answer: B

Explanation: Alcohol neurolysis (e.g. phenol injections) may reduce spasticity, but randomised controlled trial evidence of efficacy is currently unavailable. *Clostridium botulinum* toxin type A injections reduce spasticity compared to placebo, but have not been shown to improve function or quality of life. Maximal effect takes four to six weeks and lasts for 10 to 16 weeks. Side effects are uncommon but can include muscle weakness at higher doses. Indications include pain control and difficulty maintaining hand hygiene. Functional electrical stimulation has not been demonstrated to improve spasticity. Oral antispasmodic agents (including baclofen and tizanidine) only have a small effect on reducing muscle tone, and this is probably offset by the incidence of side effects. They are not commonly used. Splinting the wrist for four weeks following stroke does not reduce the risk of spasticity or contracture formation or improve function.

Reading

Scottish Intercollegiate Guidelines Network. Management of patients with stroke: Rehabilitation, prevention and management of complications, and discharge planning. National Clinical Guideline 118, 2010. www.sign.ac.uk/assets/sign118.pdf.

282 Correct Answer: D

Explanation: The risk of haemorrhagic complications outweighs the benefits of reducing venous thromboembolism with anticoagulants for most people in the first two weeks following a disabling stroke. Graduated pressure stockings have not been shown to be effective. Aspirin helps to reduce thromboembolic risk, along with adequate hydration, early mobilisation and specialised nursing care. Prophylactic dose LMWH might be used in cases at high risk, such as past history of DVT, thrombophilia or active cancer. It might also be started from two weeks after the stroke when the risk of haemorrhagic transformation is lower, if mobility remains reduced. However, in this woman's case it is likely that anticoagulation with a novel anticoagulant or warfarin would

be started after two weeks instead due to the atrial fibrillation. Intermittent pneumatic compression is an alternative option to reduce the risk of DVT, but it can cause skin damage and patient acceptance is only around two thirds in relevant studies.

Reading

Scottish Intercollegiate Guidelines Network. Management of patients with stroke: Rehabilitation, prevention and management of complications, and discharge planning. National Clinical Guideline 118, 2010. www.sign.ac.uk/assets/sign118.pdf.

283 Correct Answer: C

Explanation: Carotid artery stenting (CAS) is associated with a higher risk of periprocedural (within 30 days) death or stroke than is carotid endarterectomy (CEA). This is particularly true for people aged over 70 years. Longer-term benefits (beyond 30 days) appear to be similar between CAS and CEA. CAS avoids the need to make a neck incision and so lowers the risk of damage to cranial and cutaneous nerves. CEA can also be performed under local anaesthesia. Primary stenting has replaced the need for balloon angioplasty and may have a lower risk of complications such as arterial dissection.

Reading

Müller MD, Lyrer P, Brown MM, et al. Carotid artery stenting versus endarterectomy for treatment of carotid artery stenosis. *Cochrane Database Syst Rev* 2020; (2). Art. No.: CD000515.

284 Correct Answer: A

Explanation: Patients can return to sexual intercourse as soon as they feel ready after a stroke. There is no evidence to suggest it will increase the risk of recurrent stroke. It will not cause any significant change in blood pressure and should only affect pulse rate in a way similar to moderate exercise.

Reading

Scottish Intercollegiate Guidelines Network. Management of patients with stroke: Rehabilitation, prevention and management of complications, and discharge planning. National Clinical Guideline 118, 2010. www.sign.ac.uk/assets/sign118.pdf.

285 Correct Answer: C

Explanation: Analgesia, such as paracetamol, is the usual initial management of post-stroke shoulder pain. The rôles of positioning, EMG-biofeedback, shoulder strapping or slings are unclear. Overhead pulleys may make shoulder pain worse. Functional electrical stimulation is not beneficial for pain control. Reduced shoulder muscle activity increases the risk of developing shoulder subluxation (inferior glenohumeral joint displacement). Supportive devices, such as slings or strapping, have not been shown to prevent subluxation. Electrical stimulation of the supraspinatus and deltoid muscles has been found to improve functional outcomes when used early after stroke in combination with conventional therapy (but not for pain control).

Reading

Scottish Intercollegiate Guidelines Network. Management of patients with stroke: Rehabilitation, prevention and management of complications, and discharge planning. National Clinical Guideline 118, 2010. www.sign.ac.uk/assets/sign118.pdf.

286 Correct Answer: D

Explanation: Emotionalism is a term for emotional lability or uncontrollable laughing or crying occurring after a stroke, including laughing and crying in inappropriate situations. The natural history is to improve over several months in most people. It is a disorder distinct from depression, but symptoms may be helped by antidepressant drugs.

Reading

Allida S, Patel K, House A, et al. Pharmaceutical interventions for emotionalism after stroke. *Cochrane Database of Syst Rev* 2019; (3).

287 Correct Answer: E

Explanation: Mechanical clot retrieval can remove a blockage from a main cerebral artery and restore cerebral blood flow. It requires both an initial standard head CT scan, as all acute stroke, and an additional CT or MR angiogram study to demonstrate the vessel occlusion. Conventional cerebral angiography is then performed, under either sedation or possibly general anaesthesia, usually via the femoral artery and under X-ray guidance. A clot retrieval device, attached to a guidewire, is used to re-establish blood flow. The procedure usually follows intravenous thrombolysis unless there is a contraindication. Most commonly a stent retriever device is used; here a metallic mesh stent is expanded within the clot to trap it and allow extraction. It should be performed as soon as possible after symptom onset and probably within eight hours. There is an improved functional outcome at 90 days compared to conventional care (modified Rankin scale score 0–2, odds ratio 1.56, 95% CI 1.32 to 1.85) but no significant difference in mortality rates. Rates of intracerebral haemorrhage appear similar between groups. Possible adverse events include vessel dissection and groin haematoma formation.

Reading

National Institute for Health and Care Excellence. Mechanical clot retrieval for treating acute ischaemic stroke. Interventional procedures guidance IPG548, 2016. www.nice.org.uk/guidance/ipg548.

288 Correct Answer: C

Explanation: Guidance is to stop driving for one month after a single TIA, or a stroke from which there has been a complete recovery, and with no need to inform the DVLA. Stopping driving for three months is required for people having multiple TIAs over a short time period. People with a residual neurological deficit one month after a stroke will need to contact the DVLA. Returning to driving with a minor motor deficit may be possible, but vehicle adaptations might be required.

Reading

DVLA. Assessing fitness to drive: A guide for medical professionals. September 2019. https://assets.publishing.service.gov.uk/government/uploads/system/uploads/attachment_data/file/834504/assessing-fitness-to-drive-a-guide-for-medical-professionals.pdf.

289 Correct Answer: B

Explanation: Transient global amnesia (TGA) causes anterograde and retrograde amnesia lasting 2 to 24 hours. During an episode, the person repeatedly asks questions such as 'what am I doing here?'. No other cognitive deficits or neurological abnormalities are present, including a normal alertness level. There is no loss of personal identity. They otherwise function normally during the event. It most commonly affects people aged 50 to 70 years old. The pathological cause unknown. It can be triggered by physical or emotional stress. Recurrence is uncommon, occurring in 6%–10% of people.

Transient epileptic amnesia (TEA) has a similar mean age of onset to TGA. It more commonly affects men. The clinical features are the same as TGA but episodes tend to be shorter, lasting 30 to 60 minutes. The key difference is frequent recurrence, typically around once per month. It can occur on first waking up. It may be preceded by aura (e.g. olfactory) or associated with focal motor symptoms (e.g. lip smacking) or brief episodes of reduced consciousness. Inter-event EEG recording is usually normal. Episode frequency reduces with antiepileptic medication.

Functional amnesic states are less common and tend to affect younger people. They are linked to a stressful experience and can be associated with past depression and alcoholism. Loss of personal identity can be present. Anterograde memory may be unaffected, i.e. can learn new information such as names of attendant staff. Transient ischaemic attacks cause focal neurological symptoms. Urinary tract infections can cause episodes of delirium.

Reading

Bartsch T, Butler C. Transient amnesic syndromes. *Nat Rev Neurol* 2013; 9: 86–97.

290 Correct Answer: E

Explanation: Around 2%–8% of suspected strokes are estimated to actually be caused by functional disorders. Around 7% of acute stroke is associated with normal DWI imaging, although this is most often found with posterior circulation events. Hoover's sign has been found to have a specificity of 63% and sensitivity of 100% for functional disorders. Over the long term, only half of people recover from their disability. Specialist physiotherapy or speech therapy is valuable. Some people benefit from psychotherapy input. The presenting feature is most often limb weakness or numbness. Isolated non-fluent aphasia with preserved comprehension and naming is possible, whereas this would be unlikely to be caused by stroke disease.

Reading

Gargalas S, Weeks R, Khan-Bourne N, et al. Incidence and outcome of functional stroke mimics admitted to a hyperacute stroke unit. *J Neurol Neurosurg Psychiatry* 2017; 88: 2–6.

Jones AT, O'Connell NK, David AS. Epidemiology of functional stroke mimic patients: A systematic review and meta-analysis. *Eur J Neurol* 2020; 27: 18–26.

Popkirov S, Stone J, Buchan AM. Functional neurological disorder: A common and treatable Stroke mimic. *Stroke* 2020; 51: 1629–1635.

291 Correct Answer: E

Explanation: The patient has a lesion of the contralateral parietal lobe. The lesion is therefore in the right parietal lobe.

Homonymous quadrantanopia:

* Superior: lesion of temporal lobe
* Inferior: lesion of parietal lobe

Mnemonic = PITS (parietal-inferior, temporal-superior)
Bitemporal hemianopia:
Lesion of optic chiasm

* Upper quadrant defect >lower quadrant defect = inferior chiasmal compression, commonly a pituitary tumour
* Lower quadrant defect > upper quadrant defect = superior chiasmal compression, commonly a craniopharyngioma

---

Answers for Chapter 12: Tissue viability

292 Correct Answer: A

Explanation: Nutritional supplements should be offered to people with evidence of nutritional deficiency. Antibiotics should be used when there is evidence of cellulitis, osteomyelitis or systemic sepsis. Skin barrier creams may help with prevention by protecting the skin, e.g. from urine. A dressing that keeps the lesion warm and moist helps healing. Negative pressure dressings are not usually required. A high specification foam mattress is the standard treatment, with dynamic support surfaces used when the foam mattress is insufficient to redistribute pressure.

Reading

National Institute for Health and Clinical Excellence. Pressure ulcers: Prevention and management. Clinical Guideline [CG179] 2014. www.nice.org.uk/guidance/cg179/chapter/1-Recommendations#prevention-adults.

293 Correct Answer: D

Explanation: There is evidence from a systematic review that pentoxifylline can improve the chances of ulcer healing (alone or in combination with compression dressings). However, this is an unlicensed used of this medication. The most commonly encountered side effects are gastrointestinal in nature. There is no strong evidence to support any of the other treatment options.

Reading

Scottish Intercollegiate Guidelines Network. Management of chronic venous leg ulcers. 2010. www.sign.ac.uk/assets/sign120.pdf.

294 Correct Answer: A

Explanation:
Sharp debridement is not recommended as it may cause bleeding in friable tissue.
Specialist surgical debridement or sterile larval therapy may be appropriate following referral.

Do not clean wounds by scrubbing, which causes pain and local tissue oedema.

Do not use cotton wool or gauze swabs as these shed fibres and increase the risk of infection.

Do not use topical antiseptics.

Reviewing whether debridement is appropriate.

Natural (autolytic) debridement may be promoted by the use of specialist dressings.

Mechanical debridement (defined as removing necrotic tissue with gauze) is not recommended as it may indiscriminately remove granulation and epithelial tissue.

Reading

National Institute for Health and Care Excellence. Scenario: Palliative cancer care - malignant skin ulcer, 2021. https://cks.nice.org.uk/topics/palliative-care-malignant-skin-ulcer (accessed 9th July 2021).

295 Correct Answer: E

Explanation: The ankle brachial pressure index (ABPI) provides an index of vessel competency by measuring the ratio of systolic blood pressure at the ankle to that in the arm, with a value of 1.0 being normal. Measurement of ABPI should be undertaken by an experienced operator using validated equipment. An ABPI ratio of less than 0.5 suggests severe arterial disease. Compression treatment is contraindicated; that patient needs to be seen urgently for specialist vascular assessment. Pentoxifylline is an effective adjunct to compression bandaging for treating venous leg ulcers (off-label indication) and may be effective in the absence of compression. Antimicrobial dressings (for example silver, iodine or honey dressings) should not be used routinely. In the absence of clinical signs of infection (e.g. cellulitis, pyrexia, increased pain, rapid extension of area of ulceration, malodour, increased exudate), there is no indication for routine bacteriological swabbing of venous ulcers. All ulcers will be colonised by microorganisms at some point, and colonisation in itself is not associated with delayed healing.

296 Correct Answer: E

Explanation: Chronic lipodermatosclerosis has a gradual onset over years. Typically, non-tender legs, with sharply decreased diameter from knee to ankle, with bound-down skin are factors that help distinguish the condition from cellulitis. Whilst there is a trouble differentiating between these two conditions, they can often present together. A total of 25%–50% of patients treated for lower limb cellulitis have associated skin disease comorbidities (such as venous eczema), ulceration and oedema. These associated issues are often overlooked and mismanaged, putting strain on hospital resources, increasing the number of hospital admissions and length of hospital stay. It also puts the patient at risk of developing hospital-acquired infections and builds antibiotic resistance owing to inappropriate use. Venous stasis and eczema predispose patients to developing opportunistic infections in affected areas. Primary management of lipodermatosclerosis revolves around correction of venous stasis using compression therapy and weight reduction. Other management options include vein surgery, such as sclerotherapy and laser ablation; ultrasound therapy; fibrinolytic agents, such as stanozolol; pentoxifylline to improve blood flow; topical agents, such as corticosteroids; and analgesia, such as capsaicin, to reduce pain.

Reading

Galsinh H, Singh K, Smith L. Lipodermatosclerosis: The common skin condition often treated as cellulitis. *J Royal Coll Phys Edin* 2019; 49 (1): 41–42.

297 Correct Answer: D

Explanation: The Waterlow score permits patients to be classified according to their risk of developing a pressure ulcer—for example, a paraplegic neurological deficit, which carries a five-point value. The other options in the question are all worth three points each.

The categories of risk factors are listed below:

- Weight for height
- Continence
- Skin condition
- Mobility
- Sex and age
- Appetite
- Special risks: tissue condition and perfusion, neurological dysfunction, major surgery or trauma, medication

Reading

Scoring of Waterlow score. www.msdmanuals.com/en-gb/medical-calculators/Waterlow.htm; https://gpnotebook.com/simplepage.cfm?ID=-1684406222.

298 Correct Answer: C

Explanation: All patients should be assessed for risk of pressure ulceration at the point of admission to a hospital or care home. They should be reassessed if a major change in their condition occurs. Suitable assessment tools include the Waterlow, Braden or Norton scales. High risk is associated with reduced mobility, especially inability to self-reposition, sensory deficit of the relevant bodily area, malnutrition, cognitive impairment and prior pressure ulceration. Patients at high risk of pressure ulceration should be repositioned at least every four hours, whereas every six hours is justifiable for people at lower risk.

Reading

National Institute for Health and Clinical Excellence. Pressure ulcers: Prevention and management. Clinical Guideline [CG179] 2014. www.nice.org.uk/guidance/cg179/chapter/1-Recommendations#prevention-adults.

299 Correct Answer: B

Explanation: The heel ulcers probably result from his prolonged immobilisation during the hospital stay. Pressure ulcers remain a common problem and affect the quality of life of many patients. The majority of pressure ulcers are avoidable, and successful prevention will depend on removing or modifying the cause. Adults who have been assessed as being at risk of developing a pressure ulcer should be encouraged to change their position frequently and at least every six hours. Further pressure relief adjuncts, such as heel troughs, may be of benefit overnight but are not the primary management step. The community tissue viability team will be able to support the ongoing management. The type of pressure ulcer is not consistent with a vascular pathology. Vascular imaging would not be a first-line investigation. Provided he is eating well, a modified diet is not recommended. If a nutritional deficiency is identified, expert dietitian input would be necessary as a first port of call.

Reading

Pressure ulcers: Prevention and management. Clinical Guideline [CG179] Published: 23 April 2014. www.nice.org.uk/guidance/cg179.

300 Correct Answer: B

Explanation: Stage

I.   Intact skin with non-blanchable redness of a localised area usually over a bony prominence

II. Loss of dermis presenting as a shallow open ulcer with a red-pink wound bed or open/ruptured serum-filled blister

III. Subcutaneous fat may be visible, but bone, tendon or muscle are not exposed

IV. Exposed bone, tendon or muscle

Moisture-associated skin damage is an inflammation of the skin in the perineal area, on and between the buttocks, into the skin folds and down the inner thighs.

Index

Note: Page numbers in **bold** indicate tables.

Printed in the United States
by Baker & Taylor Publisher Services